LIGHT ON KUNDALINI

Your Lifestyle Guide to Yoga and Awakening

LIGHT ON KUNDALINI

Your Lifestyle Guide to Yoga and Awakening

by Karuna

with contributions from Kurt Johnson PhD

Copyright © 2024
All rights reserved.

This book or part thereof may not be reproduced in any form, stored in a retrieval system, or transmitted in any form by any means-electronic, mechanical, photocopy, recording, or otherwise without prior written permission of the publisher, except as provided by United States of America copyright law.

The information provided in this book is designed to provide helpful information on the subjects discussed. This book is not meant to be used, nor should it be used, to diagnose or treat any medical condition. The author and publisher are not responsible for any specific health needs that may require medical supervision and are not liable for any damages or negative consequences from any treatment, action, application, or preparation, to any person reading or following the information in this book.

References are provided for information purposes only and do not constitute endorsement of any websites or other sources. In the event you use any of the information in this book for yourself, the author and the publisher assume no responsibility for your actions. Any views or opinions expressed represent the views of the authors and do not necessarily reflect the views of the publisher.

Books may be purchased through booksellers or by contacting Sacred Stories Publishing.

Light on Kundalini
Your Lifestyle Guide to Yoga and Awakening
by Karuna
with contributions from Kurt Johnson PhD

Print ISBN: 978-1-958921-62-3
Ebook ISBN: 978-1-958921-63-0

Library of Congress Control Number: 2024945755

Published by Light on Light Press
An imprint of Sacred Stories Publishing, Fort Lauderdale, FL
Printed in the United States of America

Photography: Ryan Mastro (https://www.ryanmastro.com/), Isak Hanold, Pamela Hanson
Design: Henriqué Teixeira (https://www.htxrdesign.com/), Melanie Paykos, Sara Bercholz

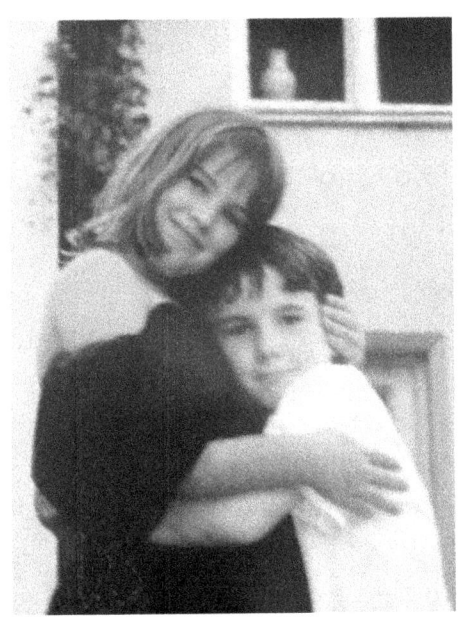

*To my dearest **Emily Laura** and **Tomas Oliver**, my children in the Divine who gave me the courage and respect to find myself, to trust, and to move into Mastery!*

ADVANCE PRAISE

In *Light on Kundalini: Your Lifestyle Guide to Yoga and Awakening*, Karuna has created the quintessential book on Yogic life. No stone is left unturned in this deep exploration that is accessible to everyone, as a wealth of compelling and enlightening wisdom and stories fill the pages, taking the reader on a journey into a truly powerful way of life. With deep dives into mantras, meditations, and everything in between, I can't recommend it highly enough.
—Steve Farrell, Co-Founder and Executive Director of Humanity's Team

Yoga is a vast topic that ultimately becomes a way of life. The journey from theory to practice, from knowledge to understanding, comes through lived experience, daily practice, and grace. *Light on Kundalini* is a living testimony of Karuna's yogic journey. It also serves as a well-articulated manual of practices led by a master practitioner. Karuna intimately shares her yogic journey as a testimony to the transformational power of Kundalini Yoga and as an invitation to others who wish to be transformed in love. Sat Nam!
—Jeff Genung, Co-Founder, Contemplative Life; Managing Director, ProSocial World

Light on Kundalini is a generous gift to the world from a truly beautiful soul. Meeting Karuna as she appears in the pages of this book will fill your mind, heart, and body with wisdom that at first glance may appear to come from many varied sources. But as you immerse yourself in this 360-degree whirlwind of teachings, stories, and practices—with Karuna as your personal guide—you will soon discover that it's the author's deep connection with the

one Source of all that allows her to interpret such wide-ranging knowledge in ways that are so very accessible, transformative, and above all, filled with love. I lovingly refer to this book as "All I really need to know about yoga I learned from Karuna."
—Kate Sheehan Roach, Co-Founder, *Contemplative Journal,* activist and editor

This book is the gift that keeps giving. Karuna has provided us with "A Yoga of Everything" guide filled with history, advice, exploration, practices, and every imaginable dimension of the Yogic lifestyle that can equip us with everything we need to awaken more deeply to our divine destiny. While reading it, I felt like I was receiving a sacred activation that inspired me to reinvigorate my yoga, meditation, and mantra practices. Thank you for this blessing, dearest Karuna!
—Diane Marie Williams, Founder, The Source of Synergy Foundation

Karuna Ji is a living, loving exemplar of the Kundalini Yoga wisdom teachings. This beautiful book captures the spirit and essence of the tradition in Karuna's unique personal style, full of love, lightness, wisdom and humour. As a general guidebook to Yoga and Awakening, it is a richly valuable resource for anyone seeking deeper truths and how to embody them in today's world.
—Ben Bowler, Co-Visioner of UNITY EARTH, World Unity Week and "Convergence" events around the world

Karuna has been a colleague and a friend for many years. Her commitments to sadhana and studentship deeply inform her teaching. Her students appreciate her humility and care, and her friendship is a balm.
—Elena Brower, bestselling author, *Practice You* and *Softening Time*

Congratulations on a powerful text. This is the testimony of a genuine Emissary of Light. This is a mature yogi who walks her talk. Karuna has trodden the spiritual path with all the lessons life brings, good and difficult, and she has allowed those experiences to teach her. The treasures that emerge here in these pages are pure gold for a seeker of wisdom.

It's a warm, welcoming book, almost conversational, that draws the reader into their own journey of Self discovery. "Come," Karuna seems to be saying in these pages, "I'll come walk with you for a while." Karuna captures, through her anecdotes, those unexpected thresholds we face in life, and presents her well tested spiritual practices here to help us navigate life.

—Swami Prakashananda, aka Rt. Rev. Chris Deefholts, Dharma Heir, Sacred Feet Yoga

TABLE OF CONTENTS

A Letter to Caroline *by Pamela Hanson* xvii
Foreword *by Denise Scotto* xix
Some Intimate Notes to the Reader xxiv
    Background xxiv
    How to Use This Book xxvi
        Sharing Our Stories xxviii
        Yoga xxx
    What Has Led You to Finding This Book? xxx
    Why a Lifestyle Guide and Daily Companion? xxxii
My Introduction to You xxxiv
    Our Childhoods xxxiv
    Our Growth xxxv
    Our Lives xxxvii

OUR JOURNEY

Finding Our Awakening 1
    Going Down the Rabbit Hole 1
        What It Means 2
        The Good News 3
        This Way Out: Assurances! 6
The Unknown of Walking Our Path 9
    Frontier Upon Frontier 10
    Step by Step 11
Failing Better and Succeeding Better 15
    Experiencing Achievement 16
    Enter Through the Narrow Door 17

OUR JOURNEY (cont.)
Letting Go of the Old and Reinventing Yourself 19
- Measuring the Steps 20
- My Rabbit Hole and My Way Out 21
- My Next Chapter 22

Radically Being You 25

LIFESTYLE
Finding Our Spiritual Practice 30
- Yoga 30
  - *History of Yoga* 30
  - *Distinguishing Kundalini Yoga* 37
  - *Elements of the Kundalini Yoga Landscape* 37
  - *The Chakras* 38
  - *Yoga Cosmology* 40
  - *Yoga and the Structure of Everything* 41
  - *Yoga and Our Human Predicament (Gunas)* 43
  - *Yoga and Finding the Birthright* 44
- Yoga Practice 46
  - *The Four Foundational Elements of Yoga – from Kundalini Yoga* 47
    - Foundational Knowledge of Body Postures (Asanas) and Hand and Finger Positions (Mudras) 49
    - Foundational Knowledge of the Breathwork (Pranayama) and Mantra 50
    - Foundational Knowledge of the Bandhas (Locks) and the Chakras 51
    - Foundational Knowledge of the Elements of Yoga Daily Practice ("Foundational," "Day to Day," and "Sessional") 53

INSPIRED MESSAGES
– with Yoga Practices

Intention 61

Our Opportunity to Connect with the Divine 63
– with Kriya for Growing Closer to the Divine

INSPIRED MESSAGES *(cont.)*

Healing Grief 65
— *with Balancing the Five Tattvas (SaTaNaMa, Kriya for Instinctual Self and Sat Kriya) and Ancient Kriyas for Healing Grief (Pittra Kriya, Shuni Mudra and Superman Pose)*

- Kundalini Yoga and Healing Grief 68
  - *Getting the Body Out of Distress* 68
  - *Balancing the Five Tattvas* 69
  - *The Ancient Kriyas for Healing Grief* 69
  - *Grief and Wisdom* 70

Becoming Zero Over and Over Again 72
— *with Kriya for Elevation*

Awakening the Ten Bodies 75
— *with Kriya for Awakening the Ten Bodies*

- Rebirthing and The International Day of Yoga (or IDY) 75
- The Ten Bodies 79
  - *The First Body Is the "Soul Body"* 79
  - *The Second Body Is Our Negative, or Protective, Mind* 80
  - *The Third Body Is Our Positive, or Expansive, Mind* 80
  - *The Fourth Body Is the Neutral, or Meditative, Mind* 81
  - *The Fifth Body Is Our Physical Body* 81
  - *The Sixth Body Is the Arcline* 82
  - *The Seventh Body Is the Auric Body* 82
  - *The Eighth Body Is the Pranic Body* 82
  - *The Ninth Body Is the Subtle Body* 83
  - *The Tenth Body Is the Radiant Body* 84
  - *The Eleventh Body Is Whole Embodiment* 84
- Global Rebirthing 85

Interior and Exteriors 88
— *Balancing, with Nabhi Kriya with Prana and Apana*

How to Stay Natural 91
— *with Sat Kriya*

Gauging Your Progress and Preventing Burnout 98
— *with Meditation Against Burnout*

- The Delight of the Frontier 98

INSPIRED MESSAGES (cont.)

   Mid-Passage 100
   What about Burnout? 102

Grace and Gracefulness in Transitions 104
   – with Nahbi Kriya

   A Flood of "Fierce Grace" 104
   The Lesson 108
   What We Don't Hear Enough About 109
   Rebuilding 110

MORE ON YOGIC LIFE

Yoga and Sound – Meditation, Mantra, and Music 113
   Meditation 114
   Sharings 117
   Mantra 119
   The Deep Mysteries of Mantra 120
   Meaning and Mantra 121
   Mantra, Personal and Communal 123
   The Esoteric Power of Mantra 125
   Kirtan 128
   Beloveds Among the Global Kirtan Community 130

Sadhana 130
   Sadhana's Many Faces 132
   Sadhana as Primal Food 132
   Sadhana as Path and Destination 134
   Sadhana in Community 136
   Kundalini Yoga Community Sadhana 137
   Personal Daily Sadhana 140
   The Importance of Personal Sadhana 141

Sustaining the Yogic Life 141

Ayurveda – Yogic Health 146
   Personality Types in Ayurveda 148

MORE ON YOGIC LIFE *(cont.)*

Body Types in Ayurveda 148
Ayurveda and Food Types 150
Reflections on Ayurveda – with Spiritual Practice 152
  My Recommendations 154
  See You in the Kitchen 157

COMMUNITY

The Wonderful Gift of Community 159
  Looking Inside Community 161
  Community, Service, and Leadership – "Seva" 164
Time and Relationships – Networks of Love 166
  We Mirror Each Other 168
Authentic Relationships 171
  Kundalini Yoga and Authentic Relationships 175
  White Tantric Practice 177
Seeing in Others What Others Can't See in Themselves 179
  Stages of Life 181
Turning the Spotlight on Yourself 184
  How that Journey Began 188
  Yoga Takes Deeper Hold of My Life 191
Finding Your Way – By Yourself and with Real Friends 195
  Finding Your Own Voice 196
Love Is the Common Denominator 200
Bigger Love – Mother Earth, Mother Gaia 204
  Cross-Overs 206

SHOULD YOU BECOME A TEACHER?

A Deeper Look 211
How Does Teacher/ Student Arise? 212
The Levels of Being a Teacher, and Teacher Responsibility 217
Companions Forever 218

"ENDING" THIS BEGINNING

Afterword by Sadhvi Bhagawati Saraswati 226

Yoga Practice Appendices 228

   1. Foundational Yoga Elements Needed for the Practices in This Book 230
      From Karuna's Yoga Manual, Foundational Guide

      Foundational Asanas, Mudras, and Other Elements 230
         Foundational Sitting Poses 230
         Foundational Standing Poses 231
         Foundational Lying (Supine) Poses 231
         Foundational General Body Actions 232
         Foundational Breathwork (aka Pranayama–Breath Techniques) ..232

   2. Revisiting the Chakras, with Fuller Details about the Bandhas (or "Locks") 235

      Chakras in Yoga Cosmology 235
      Foundational Knowledge of Bandhas (or "Locks") with Foundational Knowledge of the Chakras 235

   3. Warming Up and Tuning In & Session Closing 238

      Begin "Warm Up and Tune In" from *Easy Pose*. 238
      Warming Up 238
      Tuning In 238
      Closing a Session 240

   4. Our Opportunity to Connect with the Divine 242
      – with Kriya for Growing Closer to the Divine

      Kriya for Growing Closer to the Divine 242
         Introduction from Karuna 242
         Kriya Sequence 242

   5. Healing Grief 246
      – Balancing the Five Tattvas (SaTaNaMa, Kriya for Instinctual Self and Sat Kriya) and Ancient Kriyas for Healing Grief (Pittra Kriya, Shuni Mudra and Superman Pose)

      Reconcile, Rejuvenate, Heal, and Awaken to the Light of Your True Self 246

"ENDING" THIS BEGINNING (cont.)

- Healing Grief Practice 247
  - *Module 1: Getting the Body Out of Distress* 247
  - *Module 2: Balancing the Five Tattvas* 249
  - *Module 3: Ancient Kriyas for Healing Grief* 255

6. Becoming Zero Over and Over Again 257
– with The Kriya for Elevation

- Kriya for Elevation 257
  - *Introduction from Karuna* 257
  - *Kriya Sequence* 258
  - *Completion Message and Direction from Karuna* 262

7. Awakening the Ten Bodies 263
– with Kriya for Awakening the Ten Bodies

- Link for Free Online Instruction 263
- Awakening the Ten Bodies Elements 264
- Kriya Sequence 264

8. Interiors and Exteriors 272
– Balancing, with Nabhi Kriya with Prana and Apana

- A Kriya for Balancing, The Nabhi Kriya for Prana-Apana 272
  - *Introduction from Karuna* 272
  - *Kriya Sequence* 273
  - *6.-10. Heart Center Stretch for Healing* 275
  - *Completion Message from Karuna* 276

9. How to Stay Natural 277
– with Sat Kriya

- Sat Kriya 277
  - *Introduction from Karuna* 277
  - *Kriya Sequence* 277
  - *Completion Message from Karuna* 278

10. Gauging Your Progress and Preventing Burnout 280
– with Meditation Against Burnout

- Meditation Against Burnout 280

"ENDING" THIS BEGINNING (cont.)

11. Grace and Gracefulness in Transitions 282
– with Nabhi Kriya

- Nabhi Kriya 282
  - *Introduction from Karuna* 282
  - *Kriya Sequence* 283
  - *Completion Direction from Karuna* 285

12. Recommendations for Recipes and Music 286
- Yogi Tea: The Essential Drink for Kundalini Yoga Practice 286
- Favorite Recorded Accompaniments for Kundalini Yoga Practice 286
  - *Kundalini Morning Aquarian Chants by Jaya Lakshmi & Ananda Das* 286
  - *Albums of Choice* 287

Further Practice 288
- From the Introduction 289
- An Inspiration from Karuna 290

About the Author 293
- Teach.Yoga / Sacred U / Humanity's Stream 295
- Light on Light Magazine and Media 296
- What Karuna Wants You to Know 296

About the Contributor 297
Acknowledgments 299
Message from the Publisher 303

A LETTER TO CAROLINE

I am not sure exactly what year it was, 1978 or 1979? Boulder, Colorado, The Hill to be exact. My boyfriend, Bernard Grant, and I had a photo studio on top of a hamburger joint. We were doing tests for the Denver model agencies and had a set up in our railroad style apartment. I was doing make up, and he was shooting the photos. My make up was definitely not high end, but it seemed to work, more or less.

One day, this magical creature arrived. Her name was Carrie Pagano. Her father was the high school football coach. She was a beauty with the most wonderful aura. Not only beautiful, but funny, and fun to be with, quirky and game to try anything. Her patience and humor bonded us that first time I did her makeup; I had just had a pb&j sandwich… that's how unprofessional I was!! We did laugh about it for years. It was the beginning of a long, meaningful, and precious friendship.

We went through a lot together. She reminded me so much of my best childhood friend, Lisa Love. Not long after we met, and did a lot of photos together, she went off to Paris and early on met Lisa. The friendship was sealed; we were family. She moved to Paris but came home to visit, and we spent all our time together.

I loved her family too. We went through so much—the loss of her sister, my difficult breakup and move to Paris, marriages, divorces, having children, and losing children. We lived in London at the same time, both of us newly married and new mothers. Held each other up through those ups and downs, too.

My nickname for her was "Lucky." Somehow, she always landed on her feet. She was magnetic and attracted so much love from so many. But I now realize, it wasn't just luck. She has a magical quality about her; she always has. And she is a hard worker and an incredible friend.

I will always be grateful for the day she walked into our studio, a ray of sunshine and a breath of fresh air. I think I am the lucky one.

–**Pamela Hanson, author, Girls (2000) and Boys (2006)**
https://a.co/d/8NnaYOj and https://a.co/d/eDwK6YZ

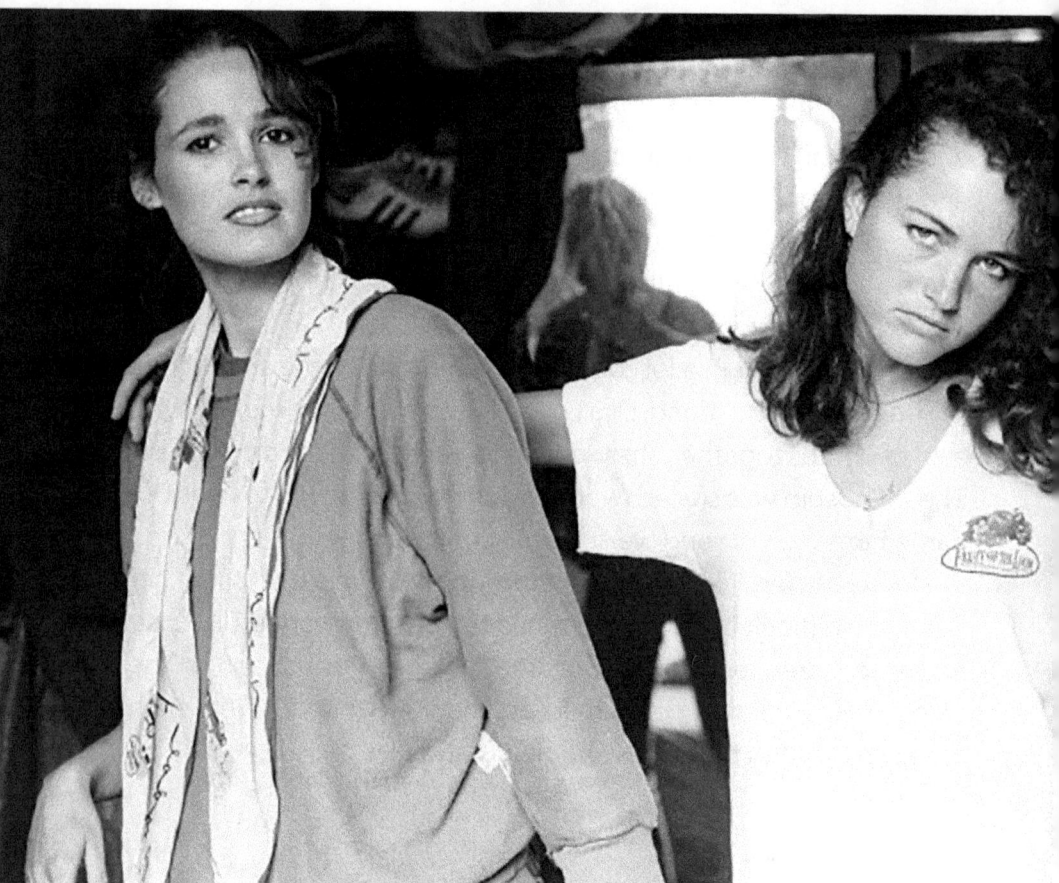

Lisa & Carrie, Paris (1979) - photo, Pamela Hanson

FOREWORD

As the Chair of the International Day of Yoga Committee at the United Nations (IDY Committee), I am delighted to write this *Foreword* to Karuna's book. For those of you who are not familiar with the IDY Committee, we are a group of Non Governmental Organizations (NGOs) in consultative status with the United Nations (UN), greater UN community members, and individual yoga practitioners.

It's been my honor to be involved with organizing and serving as MC for the official UN Observations of World Yoga Day. This has included introducing the Prime Minister of India, the Hon. Narendra Modi; the Mayor of the City of New York, the Hon. Eric Adams; the Deputy Secretary General of the UN, the Hon. Excellency Amina Mohammad; and other dignitaries as well as yoga masters. In 2023, with the Hon. Prime Minister, we created a Guiness Book of World Records for a collective yoga session with the participation of people of most nationalities. It was exhilarating!

At the same time, I've been privileged to have walked in and around the halls and conference rooms in New York UN Headquarters in the capacity as an employee working on issues concerning human rights, labor, social, and economic policy. In addition, as a leader of UN staff clubs and committees within the greater UN community, I've had the distinction of meeting spiritual leaders and yoga masters from different parts of the world, some of whom I am still in contact today.

Due to its explosive popularity and universal charm, the UN General Assembly (UNGA) adopted a Resolution marking June 21 as World Yoga Day, already some ten years ago now. A total of 177 nations co-sponsored the Resolution, which is the highest number of co-sponsors ever for any UNGA Resolution of this kind.

LIGHT ON KUNDALINI

You can read more about this from the viewpoint of the Hon. Past Permanent Representative of India to the UN in New York, Ambassador A.K. Mukerji, who accepted my invitation to write a short article for the 2019 IDY Committee Edition of *Light on Light Magazine* for which I serve as special guest editor.[1]

In supporting UN Sustainable Development Goal (SDG) 3, Health & Wellbeing, the Resolution notes how yoga, an ancient practice, relates today to promoting healthier choices and lifestyle patterns that foster good health and emphasizes a holistic approach to health and wellbeing.

While practicing yoga offers multiple beneficial gains and is an important means toward healing, developing a yoga routine also sharpens the intellect, offers a way toward inner peace, and gifts endless possibilities. Patanjali said, "A mind free from all disturbances is yoga." Swami Satchidananda, known as the Woodstock Guru, referenced this when he said, "Calming the mind is yoga. Not just standing on the head." This, my friends, is the nature of yoga 'off the mat.'

Being a decades-long meditator, I know that engaging in yoga practice gives rise to the present. Concentration while performing asanas can settle one's emotions and still the mind. And, as Vietnamese Buddhist monk Thick Nhat Hanh has said, "Meditation can help us embrace our worries, our fear, our anger, and that is very healing. We let our own natural capacity of healing do the work."

One of the most eminent yoga masters, B.K.S. Iyengar, is known for this famous quote, "Yoga cultivates the ways of maintaining a balanced attitude in day-to-day life and endows skill in the performance of one's actions." Yoga is about uniting the physical form with the emotions, the mind, the spirit, and the web of life

---

[1] https://issuu.com/lightonlight/docs/lightonlight_un_idy_2019

or the universe. Yoga helps us to better accept ourselves and the challenges life presents. As another renowned yoga master, Sri Aurobindo, explains, "The practice of Yoga brings us face to face with the extraordinary complexity of our own being."

Yoga practitioners describe how yoga is a way of life. We convey how yoga's influence is both individual and collective. As Swami Sivananda stated, "This world is your body. This world is a great school; this world is your (silent) teacher." I've had the opportunity to see the outcomes of common vision and action that benefit so many through my work at the UN and through the projects of IDY Committee NGO members. It brings to life the words of B.K.S. Iyengar when he said, "Yoga is firstly for individual growth, but through individual growth, society and community develop." By our joint efforts in service for world benefit, to quote Paramahansa Yogananda, "Humans become angels on Earth, not in heaven."

The community aspect of yoga reminds me of one of my first experiences with Karuna. We were introduced by Dr. Kurt Johnson, our mutual friend, in 2015 in Salt Lake City, Utah, where I was a speaker at various events at the 6th Parliament of the World's Religions. After meeting for the first time, a few days later, we decided to share some time together at *langar*. It just felt so right, as it connected our hearts to each other and to everyone there. Langar is a hallmark of Sikh faith. It is a tradition of cooking, serving, and eating a vegetarian meal while sitting on the floor as equals in a communal hall. All are welcome, and there is no fee to partake of the meal. The underlying purpose is selfless service which cultivates the birth of caring communities through the values of sharing, inclusion, and the oneness of humanity.

I appreciate Karuna's genuine desire to expand the evolution of human consciousness through her contribution as a Kundalini Yoga teacher/practitioner. She draws from her own life, sharing personal stories while applying the fullness of her yogic practice and its philosophy to inspire others. As an Interfaith Minister, I also value her references to other faith traditions and beliefs because, after all, as it has been said by many wise people—*the truth is one, while the paths are many.*

To use her own words, Karuna presents a 'lifestyle guide and a trusted companion.' She provides practical 'tools' while introducing the reader to one's inner knowledge and the mystical side of life. As I was reading passages of her book, I was reminded of the *Bhagavad Gita*, "Yoga is the journey of the self, through the self, to the self," and the quote by Krishnamurti, "One must know oneself as one is, and not as one wishes to be, which is merely an ideal and therefore fictitious, unreal; it is only that which is that can be transformed, not that which you wish to be."

Karuna's understanding of the cosmology of yoga reinforces how practicing yoga expands one's understanding beyond one's individual self to our bond with others and to our natural world. The values of yogic philosophy bind yoga communities and organizations together to take collective action usually voluntarily toward common goals that create a better world for everyone and our precious planet.

Be it through building water treatment systems to eradicate fluorosis, providing free education to marginalized youngsters, supplying free medical treatment in remote rural areas, or promoting a culture of peace and nonviolence, our yoga communities have made our mark. As Ammachi, Mata Amritananadmayi Devi, known as the Hugging Saint from Southern India, has stated and demonstrates, "True happiness is when the love that is within us finds expression in external activities," and "Real service is the power that sustains this world. When human beings serve nature, nature serves human beings."

Karuna's book touches upon the importance of community awareness by yogic groups. This united identity provides insight into universal responsibility and urges individuals to combine their efforts for practical outcomes to end all kinds of suffering and to accomplish seemingly impossible tasks. This rests upon the underlying values of kindness, empathy, and altruism. Buddhist monk Matthieu Ricard writes about them and the power of compassion to change oneself, our families, our communities, and our world at large: "Loving-kindness and compassion are the two faces of altruism. It is their object that distinguishes them: loving-kindness wants all beings to experience happiness, while compassion focuses on eradicating their suffering."

As I conclude, I refer to the contemporary yoga master Sadhguru who has graced us at the UN celebrating World Yoga Day and is well known for promoting the Save Soil Campaign through the ISHA Foundation. He stated, "Our lives become beautiful not because we are perfect. Our lives become beautiful because we put our heart into whatever we do."

In enjoying the pages of Karuna's book, I encourage readers to keep an open mind and an open heart. Embrace curiosity and whatever arises. Above all, be grateful for the opportunity to explore the fullness and richness of yoga.

In unity and peace,

Denise Scotto, Esq.
Chair, International Day of Yoga Committee at the United Nations
UNYogaDay.org

SOME INTIMATE NOTES TO THE READER

Background

This book came about through more than a decade of discussion about how any of us find the unique path to "our Destiny." Well-being, happiness, and an "awakened" life are our birthright, and thus our destiny, but how do any of us find our *unique* path?

This has been the consummate theme of all of my work in Yoga and inspired lifestyle for three decades, through my foundation–Light on Kundalini.

When—several years ago—I was a part of founding the *Light on Light* magazines, their companion radio series on VoiceAmerica, and annual partnership with the Committee for the International Day of Yoga at the United Nations for promoting Yoga Day worldwide, this brought this work to thousands more worldwide—as the Committee's Chair, Denise Scotto, Esq. has so generously written of in her Foreword.

But was there a need for a guide or handbook of sorts, based on all that we had learned, to further enrich and promulgate this message and this journey?

In 2019, between an annual meeting of The Evolutionary Leaders Circle in Colorado and the memorial event for our beloved friend and interspiritual pioneer Fr. Thomas Keating in Aspen-Snowmass, I sat down for a month with my friend and colleague Dr. Kurt Johnson, another interspiritual pioneer, with such a volume in mind. In daily conversations, I spoke, he transcribed, and then we discussed. The result was nearly three hundred pages of content about this sacred journey each of us has to discover our unique "Destiny." The subsequent COVID era provided the opportunity to digest and shape this material.

A lifestyle guide and trusted companion which facilitates the opening to and unique experiencing of the divine within our "every-day" lives...that is how best to describe the contents of this book. It is my message, first spoken to Kurt for several weeks on the back deck of my home beneath the 33 spectacular peaks of the Continental Divide, and then, through refining our discussions, shaped into this book, including insights and elaborations from Kurt's expertise, especially in science and Interspirituality.

Finally, some notes about attributions and about words from various languages. Regarding attributions, you will note that for some often-used "sayings" or quotations from across spiritual community, I don't provide a specific source or attribution. This is because many such oft-used "sayings" and quotations have long *lost* their precise origins and, today, are often repeated in varied versions. They are, nonetheless, staples of good, common-sense wisdom and, thus, valuable for use herein. As well, many texts attributed to ancient teachers are now simply in public domain and, regarding other historical Masters, also quoted widely (and sometimes varyingly) in diverse texts, or on the internet without detailed attributions.

Regarding "foreign" words and capitalization, we are embracing here at least four languages (English, Sanskrit, sometimes Hindi, and Gurmukhi [the root language of Kundalini Yoga]). Generally, specific words from Sanskrit, or any other non-English language, are always italicized so that they can then be fully explained. I make exceptions where the Sanskrit name has become the same (or nearly so) in English (like Chakra, Karma, Sanskrit, Ayurveda, Asana, Mudra, Bandha and many more). Further, if a word from another language has been chosen, through history, to represent a *category* in Yoga, I will sometimes also put it in quotes when it is used the first time (like the "*Gunas,*" the "*Tattvas,*" etc.), but thereafter, it will not be in quotes.

Regarding capitalization, I often use it for emphasis. For example, I capitalize Yoga and Yogic so their importance and integrity is always emphasized. I also capitalize Teacher when it is used specifically for the same reason. Also capitalized, when used as proper nouns, are Field, God, Source, Divine, and so on. Other words are capitalized by the conventions found in most religious books, like Great Wisdom Traditions, Great Masters, and so on.

I also have decided to capitalize Village, which has a special meaning in this book. It is a metaphor, for community, I use throughout—and introduce you to in my first "Intimate Note" below. We never outgrow our need to learn, and we never outgrow our need for a Village.

How to Use This Book

My hope is that every paragraph of this book can be like a really big hug—a big *welcoming* hug. I want it to be your invitation to a kind of "resort for your soul"—a place I have invited you to turn to and to "check in"—where you can take a break, relax, and reflect.

Yet, it is not just that. It is a "care-fully" architected wisdom Village, too, where you can join rest and relaxation with your deepest nature as explorer. There is much to prospect here with its many shops and storefronts, each offering different and various effects—wisdom gems, products, tools, excursions—adventures really. You won't be able to visit or to try them all at once; that will take some time. So, you'll likely want to begin by wandering around a bit and seeing what attracts you, in both the Village and the grandeur of its grounds. We never outgrow our need for learning, nor our need for a Village—a caring community in which we can actualize the fullness of our Divinity.

As you settle, you will eventually get to know the whole town—what it has to offer and where you'll find you are invited to stay awhile, and to dive in more deeply. You'll also discover there is plenty of time—because this resort is really the place of our whole existence, the setting in which you, and we, all find ourselves. It is a magical place.

There is a birthright here—a birthright about our own Awakening. Here, you'll soon discover you aren't just visiting—to relax, learn, explore—but that you have lived here all along.

Many of the "chapters" in this book are really "vignettes"—evocative descriptions, accounts, or episodes. They are like the shop and storefront signs meant to invite your interest—here, or there—and then meant to fill, and satisfy, these interests as you choose to proceed (much like the best parts of your soul-journey thus far, and I can assure you, what is yet to come).

This is why, in constructing this book, I follow the opening evocative inspirations of "OUR JOURNEY" with expositions of Yoga Cosmology in "LIFESTYLE" and then provide the spiritual practices contained in "INSPIRED MESSAGES *with Yoga Practices.*" This sequence provides you with *immediate* experiences of both inspiration and practice. Then, we proceed with further elaboration in "MORE ON YOGIC LIFE" (Meditation, Mantra and Music, Sadhana, Yogic Health, etc.) and "COMMUNITY" (Relationship with Yourself, Others, and the Earth).

This makes the book a handbook—a guidebook—about which I'll say more soon about its efficacy. In a handbook, you don't necessarily read linearly. You go to what interests you or what is needed in the moment—e.g., how to build a fire, how to pitch a tent, or how to tie this or that knot. As you do this, you not only meet your interests, or fill your needs, but you also experience fulfillment, pride, and gratification in each and every discovery, each and every new accomplishment.

In a way, it's like moving about the petals of a rose. You can move them as you like, in any direction, but, in the end, you find them all to be a part of one great whole, with every individual element—every petal–serving and enlightening that whole. That's what I want this experience to be like for you.

I hope that our shared Village–this place of real Wisdom–will be one where each house, shop, storefront, and lawn will lavish its immeasurable gifts on you and that, within each, you'll find unrestrained sacred gems, crystals–indeed talismans–of being and doing. I hope they will be, at once, of myriad colors and yet "just right" for you–"just right" for every unique occasion in your unfolding life.

Sharing Our Stories

If you expect to read this book to just learn about my story, you'll have missed the main point already. Stories have great value, especially as teaching tools and points of connection, but none of us enjoys people just rattling on about their lives or using stories to either kick up commotion or to trump others' claims and highpoints through their own, self-absorbed reports and anecdotes.

There's something deeper to story, what the great mythologist Joseph Campbell called "the hero's journey," and that's what we're interested in. We're interested in *your* hero's journey to finding a better and fulfilling life, to finding your unique destiny.

As you get deeper into exploring this Village, I–and all the shopkeepers–will, of course, be suggesting you "try this, try that" to provide guidance when you come to a puzzling fork in the road, a large boulder blocking the path, or a dark, dead-end street. That's what we're here for. The goal is to help you to change your frequency (with Yoga practice) so that you are in an expansive and quiet place–and not in a reactive one–where you no longer have the need to engage in commotion or subtle one-upmanship. This inner revolution will make life flow easier–for you and everyone around you–even when facing tough decisions, dogged challenges, or the darkest of egresses. It begins to give a sense of consistency to everything you do, no matter the circumstance.

You may even find people remarking that being around you is like "finding an oasis of peace." Following a conscious Yogic practice, mindful activities, healthy diets—yes, even new habits like vegetarianism and veganism—can create peace, quiet confidence, stability, constancy, and a life of consistency all around you.

At its heart, it's all about Yoga, and Yoga conveys "Union." So, that's the kind of life we are talking about.

Essentially, I wanted to make this book a "ready-made" toolkit for life. Each handy subtitle guides you to a vignette that contains within it both a life-lesson and a recommended life direction. As you move to the subsequent sections of the book, each will also suggest, and guide you, to a potential or specific Yogic-conscious practice. Like all toolkits, for every situation or challenge, you can just open the book, navigate to the appropriate section, and "use the right tool."

As I have said, hopefully, navigating this book will be like enjoying a rose. You can move your nose around the petals and see where you're drawn. As you explore, you will see that I often introduce things in "bigger picture" first, frequently from a life lesson or challenge with which, from your own life experience, you'll identify and be drawn to. Then, I'll recommend remedies and suggestions, not only from a wider vision but also from specific practice—real actions you can take to get real results.

Just like the depth of who we all are, the depth and breadth of conscious Yogic practice (indeed life itself!) is vast beyond comprehension. Ultimately, across these pages, you'll begin, and continue, a journey through the infinite panorama of conscious "Union" in all of its aspects. And, here within this immeasurable landscape, you'll find this book to be a trusty, true, daily companion, full of diverse tools, beacons, signals, and guidance, for developing your lifestyle with conscious practice.

Yoga

You already know that my own life-description is as "a Yoga teacher and lifestyle coach." My own name *"Karuna"* means compassion and was given to me by the Yoga Master who both embraced who I was already, and then sent me even further on my path.

So, yes! *Yoga* itself means "Union," and as you shop this wisdom Village, you will see how all the elements, advised and advertised, are part of that "whole" that comes with Yoga. All the conscious tools recommended, all the possibilities and potentials in Yoga, are tools that are part of your birthright. In the end, your birthright is what it's all about.

Particularly central and important will be the Kundalini Yoga of my core training, lifestyle, and practice. Kundalini Yoga, because it emphasizes the deeply mystical aspects Yogic spirituality, is often called Yoga's "deeper dive" and a "Raj" (royal) or "Direct Path" Yoga. I will say much more about this as our conversation unfolds.

So—whether you have come here *new* to Yoga, or as an already seasoned adept—this Village has been built for you. You can start from wherever you are and then go as far as you choose—whatever makes your heart sing.

What Has Led You to Finding This Book?

Let's now explore what has brought you to this book, why you've picked it up. There are obviously things going on in your life that have led this book to be in your hand, that made the title attractive to you. So, what is the landscape of your life right now?

It's not like it's my business to be asking you about your life—I get that. But perhaps it is my business, and potentially useful, if I tell you what was going on in *my* life when I turned to a conscious and transformative path and share my experience with you. My life was changed completely. It's important to know that you may find vital things in this book for your life. I think I can say that—assuredly from my own life-experience—if you actually adopt and absorb some or many of the ideas and visions in this book, you are lucky indeed.

I know, especially, that at first no one in their own right—or even in their right *mind*—might choose to believe that this consciousness stuff—the "S" word, the spiritual stuff—actually works; not to mention the "Y" word—the Yoga. There are just too many choices today, too many outlets, too many answers, too many choices. Sometimes, it takes a lot of life-work to reach a point of transformative change. As one great Vedic guru said, "You tend to wake up when you've gotten tired of everything else." So, even if you've already dipped into the conscious or spiritual life, and Yoga—and know the truth of what I just said above—this book may be exactly the right one to take you *even deeper*. I'm still finding books, and teachers, which do that for me.

In all the clutter in today's life—the proverbial forest wherein you may not see the trees—you don't want to miss that one unique tree, or trees, which may be the way of ascent for you. This book aims to help you find those vehicles for ascent.

So, a mutual congratulations to us for meeting here. Let's delve deeper now into the panorama of conscious transformation. In the context of Yoga, this includes not only the ancient wisdoms of our world's great religions and perennial philosophies, but also the *fact* that our bodies are *designed* as the vehicles for the conscious journey and are the very blueprints for our inevitable Awakenings. To this we will add, as well, the perspectives of modern science, psychology, diet, nutrition, and fitness.

Lastly, there is a slight of hand in all of this. One can honestly say that the wisdom of the Great Traditions, and the vehicles of Yoga, can "get you to the destination" whether you go to the left, the right, straight ahead, backwards, or even inside-out. This truth is woven into the multiple meanings ancient Sanskrit ascribes to the word *Yoga*. So often taken today as referring *only* to actions, positionings, and postures of the human body—as in much of popular commercial Yoga—Yoga of the ancients, and across the demographics our modern world's religions, actually points to, and embraces, *both* the purely passive (meditative) aspects of the path *and* also the active ones employing positioning and movement of the body.

The root of the Sanskrit word *Yoga*— "yuj"—has two, quite polar, meanings, especially because "yuj" is seldom used alone. One meaning of the root "yuj" points to the fruit of the stationery, surrendered concentration that leads to the realization of union or Oneness—"I am That" or, in the western Bible, "I am *That* I Am." This is (Anglicized) "*yuj samadhi*." But, the other meaning of the root "yuj" points to the actions, the methods, and the techniques to "join," to "connect," or to "yoke"—"*yujir Yoga*." Both of these point to there being nothing separate in the first place—the knowledge of Union, Oneness, or Divine Identity—the birthright of us all. Of course, what else could be true if nothing was "separate" to begin with?

Accordingly, we have recognized across the Yogas the "Tri-marga" or Three-fold Path(s) of Yoga—very loosely, the Yogas of devotion (*Bhakti*), actions (*Karma*), and knowing (*Gyan* or *Jnana*)—and, after these, many other variations as well. Obviously, they are all intertwined, the great Yogi Sri Aurobindo likening them as gateways into the same room.

So, this is the great journey, and the great arrival, that awaits—all to reach the same place.

Why a Lifestyle Guide and Daily Companion?

Think about it—lifestyle is, literally, how you live. Thus, lifestyle will actually *be* how you live, and the quality of that life—as it appears to both yourself, and others. A guide and daily companion means a book that is actually carried around and pulled out to consult for the purposes and needs of the moment.

It's likely that you, like I used to, live life piecemeal. Maybe you've never given much thought to how all the pieces fit together, or how they might fit together better, just for you. Or, if you have thought about it, perhaps you eventually gave up because it was just too vast, complicated, and confusing.

We can approach our lives piecemeal, or we can approach it in a way that unifies—draws together—all aspects of our lives into one concordant landscape. This should not be mysterious. This is how nature operates, what we have perennially called "the balance of nature"—a place for everything, a rhythm, a community of interactions. It's a Village as well. Such a landscape in our own lives is one of happiness and fulfillment *naturally*. It's quite self-defining.

The vignettes in this book make it very down-to-earth. Each of these life-episodes include a piece of life that you have likely experienced or had deep questions about. We share about that part of life, that part of the journey, and then offer an array of recommendations, solutions, and directions that have proved to be fruitful and "right" in our own experience and may work for you.

So, just like a guidebook for exploring, cooking, camping, hiking, birdwatching, or whatever the case, you'll be able to scan these subtitles and key in on the ones that are relevant to you in this or that moment.

Then, once you've gotten the hang of the whole landscape, and a sense of *your* landscape, you'll be able to decide where you want to land for this day or that, at this time of your life or another—just like deciding what landscape you'd like on a trip—waterfalls today or forests tomorrow—whatever your choice. We can make this all work for you.

MY INTRODUCTION TO YOU

from Karuna

In order for this offering to be useful to you, it is important that I look back a bit and tell you how the journey reflected in this book—combined with all the activities (the conscious practices) it recommends—was pivotal to me in actual life and led, eventually, through real transformation, to a happy, fulfilled, and manifest life.

As I've said, the whole purpose of this book is about *lifestyle*, about how you may decide to live. I've already told you that the greatest discoveries in my transformative path were from the gifts of Yoga. You may already be familiar with Yoga—at least as it is known in the West—or perhaps not. I'm not going to over-emphasize the Yoga at first, because it came into my life as part of my discovery of my own conscious transformative path as well, but emphasis on it will grow and grow in this book, just as it did for me in my own life. But we'll start with consciousness and the desire we all have for a quality life, a life of freedom and safety and the pursuit of real happiness.

Our Childhoods

My journey, like yours and so many millions, began when I was a child. Like you, I had those moments out under the stars, or looking at a sunset, and asking the perennial questions: Who am I? Where did I come from? Why am I here? What is my future? Like you, when I heard music, I wondered why I was so moved and why it affected me so deeply. Why did I want to move my body with it? And then there was the mystery of *Love*. What is *that*? And what about *change*? What is up with *that*?

We are all novices growing up, and we often do not come across that many guidebooks in our early years. Like you, especially in my younger years, there were many detours and blind alleys. There were so many enticements, so many stories, so many promises. Also, when we are younger, there is often so much responsibility taken for us by others, not necessarily ourselves.

And so, I am sure you remember those first sobering moments after your younger years when you encountered adolescence and then "growing up." You remember those moments of reckoning when you were first by yourself. Perhaps it was in college, in high school, or in your first job. Those were the moments when you realized "the buck stops here, and it's up to me what I make of this life." That is often when the crossroads of life appear, and, at those crossroads, we can either go on unguided and unaided for a long time, or we may, by luck (or more likely grace), begin to find the guiding points on our soul's compass, our real north stars.

Likely as you were reading this you did an instantaneous scan of your whole life. I know I did when writing it. For many of us, life has likely been a rather jagged path, perhaps even an arduous collapse and rebuilding (as in a "12-step" journey). For others, maybe it's been smooth and full of luck. Whatever our stories, we have met here, in the current "here and now" with this book in your hand– discovering your destiny. Perhaps we can begin to assess together what we know from our inner compasses, our north stars, or what Divine Guidances have Intervened.

Our Growth

It may not surprise you that my transformative journey began with music. Over forty years ago, by what would appear to many as sheer coincidence, and a business friendship, I was delivering flowers to a funeral. This was a funeral in the Sikh tradition, and while I was placing the flowers, the musicians were practicing. This was the most beautiful music I had ever heard. I found out later it was the music of the Kundalini Yoga tradition—harmonium, *veena* and *ektara* (stringed instruments of India), *tabla* (one-sided drums), *mridanga* and *pakhawaj* (two-sided drums), flutes, *karatalas* and *talas* (cymbals), and voice. Although I didn't know it then, I understand now that these musicians work from the Heart Chakra and on up through the Crown Chakra through the "Tenth Gate" to raise the frequency of any environment. I was so profoundly moved by this experience that I explored a Yogic path.

As I later pursued Kundalini Yoga in depth, I realized that it was the music also that would free my mind in relation to the asanas (postures) so that I could flow into them and not be resistant as I developed my Yogic practice. I understand now that many things in me before this time had been resistant. What a gift (chance? Divine intervention?) to have been led to this crossroads in my life. As I would cultivate this practice in my deepest private time, I came to sense grandeur—simple, but grand: "I am a human being, and I can begin to *deeply* understand connection to the divine."

Duality—any sense of separateness—began to leave me. I was no longer interested in just trying to "get" things, and believe it or not, prosperity and opportunity began to come *to me*. When my heart was open, I discovered I was more still and present, letting go and receiving the processes of life organically rather than pushing. In the practice, I found increasing steadiness and what is called the "simran flow" (a Sanskrit term meaning "the sense of highest aspect") of meditative mind. *"Simran" also* means "recognition," and I recognized quite soon that I was a Bhakti Yogi, a yogi of love and devotion.

I ended up taking all the Kundalini Yoga courses I could find, and I also met a mentor teacher. One day, she looked at me and said, "Your destiny is to become a teacher." I instantly believed it, and within two weeks, I was on a plane once a month to go to a teacher training program. Of course, no one can just complete a teacher training program and think they are suddenly a Master Teacher. That is a long, and life-long, process, and one not set out for making claims about achievement. It is others who call Masters "Masters," not ourselves. Each of us begins by practicing as a student. It was the same for me. Continuing daily practice, we polish and deepen the essence that is already our birthright, our divine nature. And, it naturally awakens. It's built in. We move out of ego and identification with the past. We move into the dynamic freedom of who we really are. Remember, change your story, and you change *You*. It's the opportunity that Yoga practice gives us to become our True Selves.

Our Lives

Life is a living change, a new day every day—forever actually. In this grandest sense, the basic purpose of life is just to be human and to deal with life as a human being. And this is a life full of relationships and inter-relationships. Here, the ideal is balance. Remember the wiseman saying, "Don't become bitter so that someone will throw you away or so sweet that someone will devour you." There is wisdom in this Middle Way that all the great traditions have taught. Also, there is nothing in the Middle Way that distracts from the high and singular points of focused practice that also unfold with the Yogic life.

Another part of Yogic life that has been significant to me is learning about communication. The great traditions often refer to the array of communication involved in life as "transmission"—since communication is reaching between one point to another. There is transmission of the written or verbal word; there is transmission through all the avenues of art; there is transmission through the resonant Presence of being itself; and, most of all, there is transmission with the Divine. Some seers say that "meditation" is when you are inquiring about communication and that "contemplation" is when something answers. A relational dialogue begins.

I often have reflected on why transformational music is so important and have come to realize that it is because it stokes the energy from Heart Chakra on up through the Crown Chakra to infinity. This is in contrast to the other types of music which stimulate energy in the lower chakras. All forms of music have their place. There is a universal rhythm to truly transformational music. Other music that is simply more physical or mental can interfere with the deeper cosmic rhythm. Commotional, emotional music can evoke a way of being which can conflict with the natural essences of you by misunderstanding what the heart is saying, simply because it creates a dynamic that is at odds with the steady, universal groove emanating from the Divine around us and within our inner being. Transformational music aligns with the innate rhythm of the sacred around us and within us, bringing us back into harmony with our deepest, Truest Selves, becoming one with the natural rhythym of the Self and Gaia.

Yoga and Yoga classes are about elevation, so you need the protection of the proper combination and permutation of silence, words, sounds, and movement to push you through. You need a rocket to launch a space shuttle, to get it into orbit and outer space where it can take care of itself. Yoga's relationship to transformation is the same way, and music is a part of that propellant which launches the person from within.

For me, the Yogic lifestyle has included everything—sharing understandings of nature, of food, of self-sustained living, of sound and touch, of relationship, of community, and of immersion in *every* mystery and dimension of Being—and *all* is in service to community. This is, as is often said, the vast embracing landscape from "I" to "We" to "Us" to "All of Us."

Concluding my personal note, looking back on it—it appears that, in this journey from student to teacher, there was a wisdom to it all. As our lives further unfold, what are we going to do, and how are we going to serve? How can we serve if we have nothing to offer? So, in offering this book to you, I acknowledge the depth and gift of this practice and what it has given to *me*: a life where I am close to my own happiness and spirit—healthy, rested, and living in a peaceful environment. This is the life and state of being that I wish for you—and that you not only realize it for yourself but also are able to offer the same freedom and grace to all others.

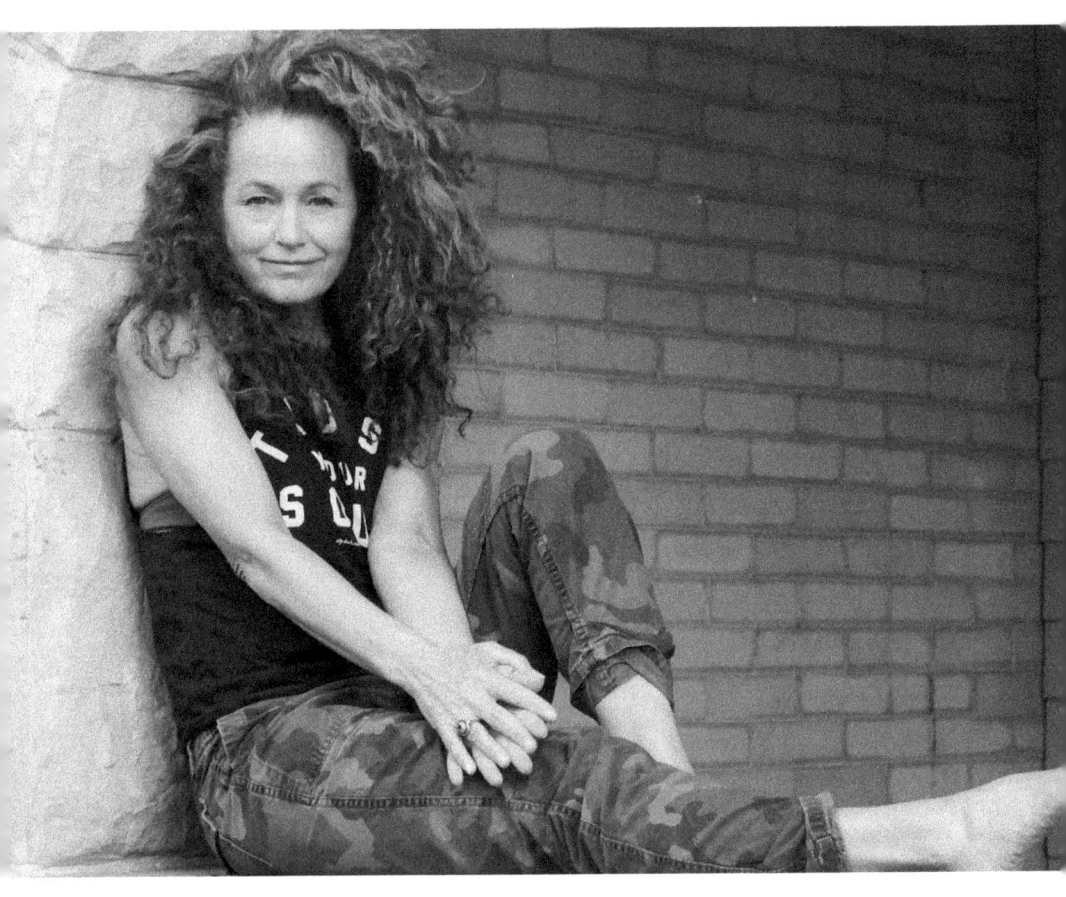

Street Clothes

OUR JOURNEY

FINDING OUR AWAKENING

Going Down the Rabbit Hole

If you are taking your life seriously right now, contemplating your path— perhaps even your destiny—your life as the truly epic journey down that infamous rabbit hole in Lewis Carroll's *Alice in Wonderland* may seem a worthy metaphor. It's a journey into the unknown. Your commitment to that unknown is what has brought you here, so I commend you for that and welcome you.

Let's talk about the rabbit hole first. As you remember: Alice sits on a riverbank on a warm summer day, drowsily reading over her sister's shoulder, when she catches sight of a White Rabbit in a waistcoat running by her. The White Rabbit pulls out a pocket watch, exclaims that he is late, and pops down a rabbit hole. Alice follows the White Rabbit down the hole and comes upon a great hallway lined with doors. As the story unfolds, all hell breaks loose: all the fascinations—the tea party, the Cheshire cat, the Gryphon— juxtapose all the dangers—the King, the Knave, and the Queen wanting to cut off Alice's head. But just as it seems she is going to die, she awakens in the arms of her loving sister, realizing it is all a dream. Alice is safe and sound and simply goes to tea.

"Down the rabbit hole" is a metaphor for entry into the unknown. It's the journey that I have made and that we're all making. And, like

Alice, in the end, we will awaken in the arms of the beloved and go to tea.

But there are tools that can make the journey very different than the one in Alice's story in wonderland. Could you imagine how different Alice's journey would have been if she were given more direction than "Drink Me" or "Eat Me," or would have been given the royal court protocol for the Queen of Hearts? She might not have been in as much danger or confusion if she had more knowledge of the situation and her surroundings. With more solid guidance, she might have woken up much sooner without her own head being at so great a risk!

Therein lie the gifts of Yoga—detailed practices and techniques to support the health and well-being of Yogic lifestyle. As many guru-teachers say, having these techniques is the express train to Awakening—something Alice did not have.

As you look through the landscape of this book—and explore the metaphorical shops and storefronts in this Village prepared for you—you'll see we'll discuss the invitation to Awakening first—awakening to your birthright for a life that is happy, healthy, and, yes, even holy.

What It Means

Let's first take a look at the multiple meanings of "going down the rabbit hole" and why they are so apt—not only to the journey of the consciousness, the journey of the spiritual life to Awakening—but also to our pursuit and assembly of the actions and techniques that hasten that journey: the gifts of Yoga. There are multiple parts to the plot of the rabbit hole that we—that you—have decided to go down: First of all, there is the *jumping in*! Then there is the question of what happens when you do? And, lastly—once you *have*, what then?

If you are on a life-searching path right now, it's probably safe to say that you have been at the gates of the rabbit hole already or likely might not have picked up this book. So, let's explore. Let's start with some random varied meanings of "going down the rabbit hole":

- a metaphor for something that transports you (wonderfully or troublingly! and either willingly or unwillingly!) into a previously unexperienced, even surreal realm;
- a metaphor for something deeply engrossing, and thus long and drawn out;
- a metaphor for a period of chaos or confusion and the seeking of a solution for it; or
- a metaphor for a deeply complex, difficult, or even bizarre situation to which the pursuit of an answer or solution can actually lead to other questions, problems, or pursuits.

Quite a tangle, right? Yet, we have all gone down rabbit holes, or simply found ourselves in them. In fact, the search for answers to the deeply spiritual questions—"Who am I?" "Why am I here?" "Where am I going?"—seem nearly certain to offer a rabbit hole. In fact, it's probably safe to say that if you weren't in a kind of rabbit hole already, you likely might not have picked up this book.

The Good News

So, here is the good news. Another fitting title for the conscious, spiritual, or Yogic enterprise (and the specific practices and tools you may pick up), certainly for Kundalini Yoga, would be: "THIS WAY OUT." How many times in your own life have you welcomed seeing that sign, showing an arrow and the words "This Way Out"?

So, what are the elements of "This Way Out?" That is what this book is about. Well, first off, they are diverse—because this cosmos is diverse. Everyone knows that when you get lost, by definition, you have no signposts, no compass readings, nor landmarks that help you to understand where you are. You are lost in a diverse landscape, and discovering the ways, markers, and directions forward requires concerted detective work. We might liken it to a maze where every corner requires some detective work to decide which way is going to help you to find your way home. Thus, in finding your way out, it's fair to say that all the decisions you will need to make are diverse indeed. And, if you were going to have tools at each stage of solving your whereabouts in the maze, these tools would be diverse as well—solving this puzzle, solving that puzzle, reaching this threshold, reaching that threshold—step by step.

But with the tangle of us being lost in the puzzle of life, in our consciousness, or identity of who we are—the perennial questions of Who am I? Where did I come from? Where am I going?—there is something very different at play. What that is is what the Great Traditions and the Great Masters call our True Nature, our Buddha Nature, our Christ Consciousness. This means that the great discovery in the predicament of being lost is that the compass, the map, has been in our pocket all the time—and it is Real.

Imagine yourself lost, as noted above, and then discovering the compass, the map, has been your pocket the whole time. Well, you would start to work with it. You could discover the clues you need and proceed step by step. But, this is only completely true in the physical landscape of being lost. The consciousness landscape, the inner landscape, is one beyond space and time. Here, it is a different matter and opens up very paradoxical possibilities. If the maze you are lost in is a physical one, you will certainly need detective work, clues, and incremental victories to find your way forward, even once you have found the map and compass in your pocket. But in the maze free of space and time, why not just jump out of the maze altogether?

It is possible, but it's not everyone's path. Awakening, that big word for finding "The Truth," "your birthright," "your Freedom," and "your Fullest Well-Being"—and it's *all* True—can be incremental, step by step, or sudden and catastrophic (catastrophically good!). It can be many small glimpses added together; it can be big jumps added together, or even one big jump. I mention this now because it is the paradoxical nature of getting out of the rabbit hole or This Way Out. You will find an amazing story about this later in this book—in the chapter "Failing Better and Succeeding Better." Sometimes, the "tangle" involved in waking up makes no apparent sense, but the result is always the same.

India's famous saint, Ramana Maharshi, gave the example of how Jesus of Nazareth taught about this paradox in his Parable of the Workers in the Vineyard. Perhaps, Ramana said, it is the most little understood of all of Jesus' parables. In the parable, Jesus notes that the workers in the vineyard were paid the same amount if they worked all day or only worked a minute. What he meant allegorically was that the result of spiritual "labor" or practice, Awakening, was all the same, whether you worked a minute or a lifetime to enter into that state of being.

This helps us to understand the paradoxical languages of Great Masters when they say things like: "we are the ones we are looking for," "our destination was where we started from; we had always been there," "we end up on the other side but don't know how we got there," "swallow the ocean in one gulp," or, in the case of the rabbit hole, "don't crawl out of the hole; simply jump out of it" or "stop the search." A few quotations like this cannot exhaust the abundance of this kind of wisdom from what our Wisdom Traditions call Great Masters. Books and entire careers of spiritual teachings by others following in their footsteps have all simply said the same thing. Ramana Maharshi himself said, according to some, "There is nothing new; we simply run across it again."

Ramana also told the story of the meaning of "the narrow door" as spoken by Jesus of Nazareth and recorded in the Gospels of both Matthew and Luke: "Enter by the narrow door that leads to life." If you are living in a purely "magic-mythic" view of reality, where you think someone has to do something for *you*–to "save" you–you will think the "narrow door" is the belief in this or that Guru or Messiah–a "ticket to heaven," so to speak. But that is not the meaning. The meaning is what we take up in the chapter right after this one: "The Unknown of Walking Our Path."

If we are speaking of the surety of This Way Out and acknowledging that your emergence into freedom may be incremental, in small steps, or big steps–or even all at once–there are assurances from the Great Masters that guarantee us that whatever the rabbit hole, and whatever the twists and turns of the stories applied to it, we will find our way out. These are certain assurances I can give you "this early in the game" to give you confidence on the way. After all, as another Great Master said, "Remember, we are playing a fair game."

The truth of the matter, and the truth of such paradoxical language, is the paradox of our own nature. We are two things at the same time. We are Divine and human at the same time. The way out of the rabbit hole is guaranteed–we just may not know how it will unfold–as the young man in the chapter "Failing Better but Succeeding Better" surprisingly discovers.

This Way Out: Assurances!

Nisargadatta Maharaj is one of most revered teachers in the modern Vedic era, famous for his iconic book *I Am That*, which

I quote from below. Wherever you go on this journey into Yoga you'll find him being honored, and quoted, with the assurances that I give you below.

First, about the personal journey and that no one initiates you, you initiate yourself:

- "Your own self is your ultimate teacher. It is only your inner teacher that will walk with you to the goal."

On spiritual discipline, the word spiritual practice speaks for itself:

- "What is wrong with striving? Striving itself is your real nature." "Even effort is a part of it." "When effort is needed, effort will appear."

On Yogic practice, everything you get from Kundalini Yoga is already inside yourself:

- "Yoga is the work of the inner self."

On Awakening:

- "You are the Self, here and now."

So, the Great Masters, revered by entire spiritual traditions, guarantee you that you are Divine Nature itself and that you can achieve the sense and knowledge of this nature that will serve you in all the levels of your life, and experience, here on planet earth. Not a bad deal!

And of the path they say:

- "Karma [the laws of cause and effect] is the law that works for righteousness; it is the healing hand of God."

LIGHT ON KUNDALINI

This is about your birthright—so it has been best to start with making sure you understand that promise. Further, let me say that Kundalini Yoga is considered a "Raj" Yoga, of which I will say more later. "Raj" refers to royalty, and, you remember, royalty is often carried on a "litter," a distinct kind of transportation. This is also why Kundalini Yoga is also considered to be a "Direct Path" Yoga.

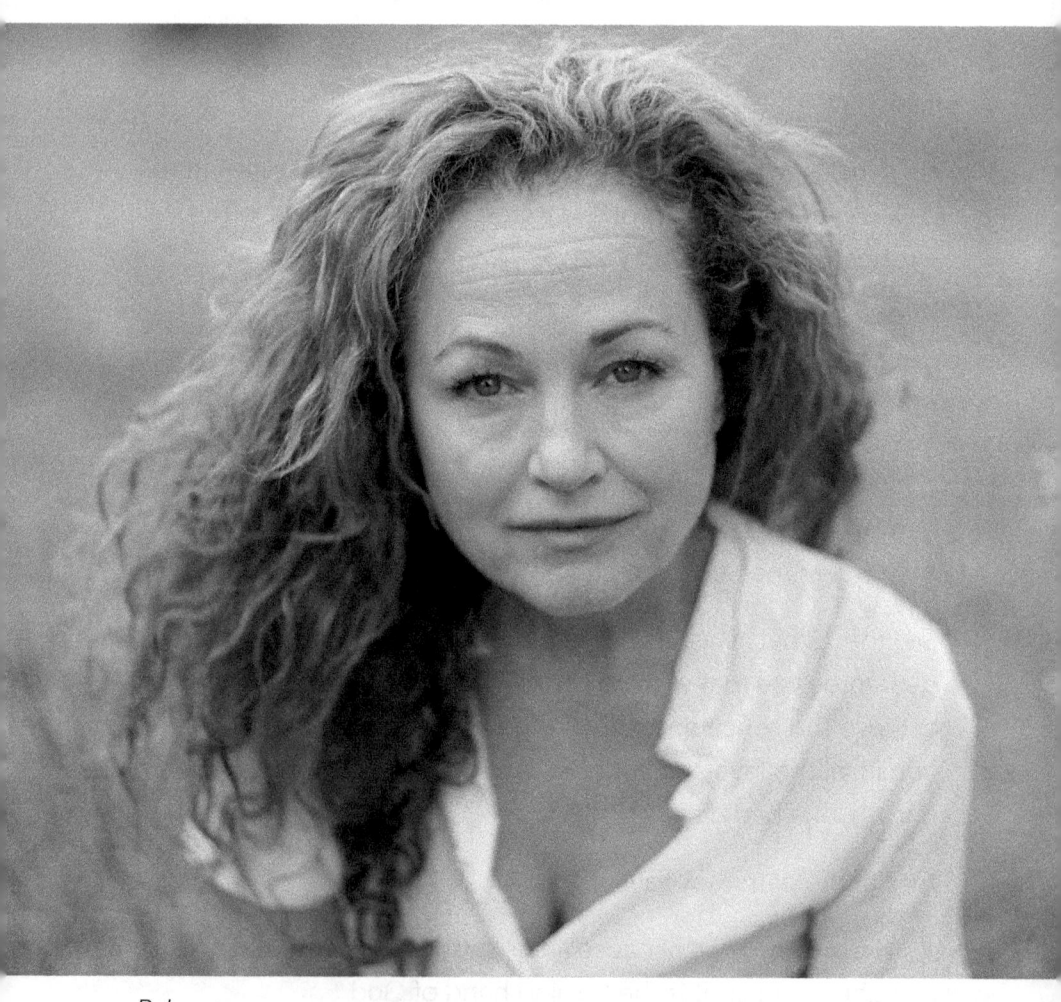

Balance

THE UNKNOWN OF WALKING OUR PATH

Going down the rabbit hole is a captivating metaphor for entry into the unknown. Rabbit holes are startling and extraordinary because they are unforeseen, and, in the experience, we have nothing to compare them to. They are entirely new, with no reference point. Such situations can be disorienting and disconcerting and can lead to us to act in a very confused manner. What do any of us do in situations that are entirely new and unfamiliar to us? And why do such situations arise, often throwing us off our paths that seemed so certain?

Such situations are common enough in life—especially when we are already making a turn, at a crossroads, contemplating or questioning a direction—because the practice of life itself is always taking you from frontier to frontier. The word "frontier" actually means a place not seen before. That word—"frontier"—and "pioneer" are connected in a deep way. Life is an unfolding of frontiers, and you are the pioneer—"a person who is among the first to explore or settle a new country or area"—actually trailblazing for your own life.

Here is where we gain courage, more deeply grounded senses of direction, and what interspiritual pioneer and monk Br. Wayne Teasdale called "mature self-knowledge." Spiritual teacher Robert Adams, author of *Silence of the Heart*, referred to this emerging deeper inner knowledge as "the current that knows" and finding the sense of that current within yourself. He likened it to that "median line" on an oscilloscope which, no matter how scattered and up and down the oscillations around it, remains steady and secure.

My prediction is that, as you enter your Yogic journey, you will suddenly have this experience within of "the current that knows." As stated in the Chrisitan mystic classic *The Cloud of Unknowing*:

"It is naught else but a true knowing and feeling of ourselves as we are."

Frontier Upon Frontier

One thing you will notice as you take up your conscious journey, your spiritual pioneering, is your constant discovery of new frontiers.

Kundalini Yoga, this journey being offered to you, provides a landscape, a cosmology, in which you will make constant new discoveries, understand things you didn't understand before, and be transported into endless new revelations. It will give you a deep sense of how the world is put together and also how you fit in. Remember—this is what I promised you when I invited you into "the Village." It will be a beginning of your deep sense of knowing—one that will, truly, "make sense."

You've undoubtedly noticed, especially in these recent times, that humans seem to love beliefs, creeds, dogmas, slogans, even conspiracy theories. Psychologists say this is because humans like things that are "easy to understand" and "easy to repeat." Scientists say it's also because such simplifications often have a short term "adaptive value"—they help you feel better, or even sometimes simply survive, in a short run situation. The problem is that such shortcuts, if not really wise and true, always eventually dead end. I am sure you have had this experience in your life. I know I did. I had to figure it out, and Yoga, which is experiential, not something you are told is true, was key.

The point of this is to tell you that your journey into Yoga will not be one of slogans, creeds, dogmas, or dead-ending stories. It will be one drawn from your own experience. Thus, a wise Teacher says, "Don't just believe what I say; test if for yourself and find out yea or nay." Yoga is meant to enter into and test out, for deepest inner self and to see how *you* experience it. Then you draw your own conclusions and make your own maps. You find that core experience of truly owning your own experience, because you have created it yourself, step by step.

This is why the conscious spiritual pursuit of Yoga itself is referred to by the ancients as a "science." Science, by definition, has four qualities, and they are also qualities that I'm sure you would want in your own life: testability (try it and see for yourself), repeatability (make sure that what you're trusting can happen over and over), predictability (if *this* is true, than *this* must follow) and veracity (the ability to explain things). You will find this is true when you take up the specific sequential practices (*Kriyas*) of Yoga. You will be able to gauge your progress by these classic criteria of science step by step. In a later chapter, I offer more specific insights about "Gauging Your Progress..." and accompany them with a specific, recommended Yoga practice.

Step by Step

Let's apply this now to the zigs and zags or our own journey, the "unknowns of walking our path." Today's modern synthesis, embracing both modern science and the deepest understandings of our Wisdom Traditions, tells us we are destined to go through five key steps in our transformative process. As a testament to evolution, it's interesting that these five steps have emerged mostly in the last ten years. The first started with Ken Wilber distinguishing between "Waking Up" and "Growing Up." There is a wonderful video on this that Ken narrated for me and my colleagues at the "Crestone Convergence" event in 2017. You can find it at YouTube by searching "Coming Together at the Crestone Convergence."

In a nutshell, as Wilber has now made a classic insight, "Waking Up" –spiritual Awakening, has been with us for millennia, ever since there was a Buddha or other enlightened Teacher. But it has not changed the world. It must be coupled with "Growing Up," the rising of humanity through stages of development to where it is truly capable of creating a world that reflects the high values and vision of Awakened consciousness. According to Wilber, true "Growing Up" has only become possible in perhaps the last 150 years, with what we now know from modern science and technology.

We *could* build that world that reflects "Waking Up," but it is a massive task—and yet one we must embrace. Wilber and colleagues, Dustin DiPerna, and others, then added "Cleaning Up" and "Showing Up," and my colleagues Kurt Johnson, Jude Currivan, and others added "Linking Up" and "Lifting Up." In a publication for the 2018 Parliament of the World's Religions in Toronto, Canada, my *Light on Light* publication defined them this way:

Waking Up (to our divine nature, our full moral capacity),
Growing Up (creating a world that reflects these heart values),
Cleaning Up (healing, reconciliation, shadow work),
Showing Up (activism and speaking truth to power),
Linking Up (creating cooperative and synergetic work together), and
Lifting Up (co-energizing and co-inspiring).

Think about these in your own life. I am sure a lot of bells will go off regarding what you've already been doing, or what you are looking for. They have become known as "the Ups" and, during the COVID lockdown, framed a week-long online event from all my friends at UNITY EARTH (https://unity.earth/) called "The Up Convergence." As you have probably realized, the whole world has to go through these steps, and it certainly has to begin with individuals, like you and me, doing it.

This is the journey that is out ahead of you. But let's make it more specific now in the context of why I've written this book and why you've picked it up. This is because I'm confident in what you'll find here. And I'm confident you'll learn this delicate mastery of what is known and what is unknown as you navigate your path. Again, as the anonymous author of *The Cloud of Unknowing* says:

> "When you first begin you find only darkness, as it were a cloud of unknowing. You don't know what this means except that in your Will you feel a simple steadfast intention reaching out toward Source. Reconcile yourself to wait in this darkness as long as is necessary, and still go on longing after It."

But we can do better than even the longing. We can step into the practice, confident that it will take us along step by step. Our tools for getting out of the rabbit hole—experiments, investigations, explorations, practices—are very specific, and they work. In the Village I have invited you into, you will find you can't stand in a shop, just looking, forever. You'll need to pick up some tools and follow that current within you. Everything I have said above about the general journey, about the conscious and spiritual enterprise, applies to all the available tools as well. You will master them step by step.

Just like with any other skill you have acquired in your life, be it in athletics, music, or career, these have come step by step, and in each case, the same steps apply: Waking Up, Growing Up, Cleaning Up, Showing Up, Linking Up and Lifting Up.

It seems to be one of the facts of our current Age that the inner knowledge from the ancients, as in the wisdom and techniques of Yoga, is meeting with the scientific knowing and technology that can create the world that the Heart wants to see. This is what is meant, at the global scale, by connecting the "Waking Up"–the deep inner knowledge–with the "Growing Up"–the determination to behave accordingly and to build a world that reflects those profound inner values discovered by the inner spiritual work.

The same is true of our own personal journey–reflecting the ancient saying "As above, so below"–the journey in which, just like for the world, your life is both "dreaming it" and "doing it."

FAILING BETTER AND SUCCEEDING BETTER

I'll bet that, if you look back at your life, you may see at each twist and turn that you did a little bit better each time and that—even if a particular chapter appeared as a "failure"—it was often, in retrospect, still for the better. "A learning experience" and "the silver lining on a cloud" are things we are all familiar with.

My twists and turns, moving from Colorado to Paris, Paris back to New York, New York to London, London to Colorado, Colorado to L.A., and back to Colorado, now appear much that way to me, especially because it was during that time that I found my Yoga practice and established my Yoga lifestyle. Each time, I was getting better. And each time, I was cementing healthier and healthier relationships.

In that process, forgiveness and reconciliation are so important. They are like the "red light" and "green light" of us moving forward. So, at every turn, try to make sure that you are "good" with your loved ones, are able to forgive, and can become a real friend to your relatives and that everyone is ready for a new start.

And, on your journey, you do get little "signs" about when it's time to go—or move on—to a next step. Often these signs resonate deeply from things in your past. When I was tinkering with leaving London for Colorado, I saw a girl get on a horse—bareback. For some reason, I said to myself, "That's me...I want that again." And when I made the decision to really make that move, my deepest inner roots supported me. It was no longer just something haphazard. Leaving somewhere happy is paramount. Like they say, "Never make decisions in a bad mood." And, what I see now is that—increment by increment—my Yogic practice and lifestyle also were taking their place as sturdy pillars for my life.

So, these are the odd twists and turns of "what's best for you" and how you learn to discern things. Everything keeps changing for the better. I guess this is a testimony to the author who coined the term "failing better" in a book titled *In Defense of Lost Causes*. We can feel like we, or situations, are a "lost cause" sometimes, but it is often part of a much bigger picture.

Experiencing Achievement

One thing that Yoga practice gives you is a container in which you can experience achievement—and especially achievement that is seen by, and celebrated by, your deepest inner self. So often, our lives have been full of others—and ourselves—not knowing real joy. That potential joy is overridden by being just in a story, or having that habit I've mentioned of thinking we have to trump another's story, anecdote, or complaints with our own.

For many who have lived in *that* world, and often felt invisible, the exhilaration of small achievements is a whole new frontier. In the practice of Yoga, you can find your gem each day, your diamond in the ruff, and keep feeding the inner polishing of that diamond week after week.

Achievement is actually a collective thing. Think of celebrities for instance. No one is a celebrity unless we make them one. When we celebrate the achievement of a sports or entertainment hero, we actually are identifying with their achievement. Brain studies show that the same parts of the brain light up when we are watching someone do something as when we are doing it ourselves. So, we wear our sport hero's numbers, or the names of our entertainment heroes, on sweaters, T-shirts, and the like. It is such a powerful stimulus that millions of dollars are made every year by selling such paraphernalia.

Scientists also say this trait is one of the major things that distinguishes us humans among all of our ape cousins. We love to share, and we love to teach. When a chimpanzee or a bonobo experiences something unique, sometimes they relate it, sometimes they don't—more often the latter. And even if they do share it, they seldom share it more than once. But when humans, even human children, experience or find something that fascinates, they want to share it right away. Scientists believe it is this "urge to teach" that has made humans the builders of so many things. There is no other animal that rivals humanity in that trait.

This is where there is an amazing convergence between Yogic practice, Yogic lifestyle, and the natural convergence of community—the Village we have been speaking of. This is why so many persons living a Yogic lifestyle profess to have a very deep happiness and often recount, with gratitude—and humor as well—the twists and turns that "got them there."

Enter Through the Narrow Door

One particular story comes to mind that is worth repeating. This is the one I told you was coming. It's about a young American man who went to India and made the mistake of thinking he could make a fast buck by selling drugs. He was caught and sentenced to twenty years in prison. In his twenties, this meant incarceration at least until his forties. He was put in a prison where there were barracks surrounding a large, rather vacant, prison yard. His first years there were miserable, and he was often mistreated because of his different ethnic background.

One day, he learned that he could take seeds from fruit trees at the edge of the prison yard and plant them *in* the prison yard. So, with nothing else to do, he focused on planting, watering, and nurturing these seeds. At first, it was a curiosity to the other prisoners and the guards, so they didn't bother him much. They treated him more like an outcast or a recluse. But soon, the trees started to grow and bear edible fruit, and, in sharing the fruit, he created not only a welcome treat for his fellow inmates and guards, who loved to eat the fruit, but also a communal spirit.

Some ten years into this process, he sat back and had a realization—truly an Awakening realization. He saw that the natural and cosmic flow that he had created from his unhappiness and desperation had morphed into something that was not only good but also was bringing real happiness to others. He realized that he had "Awakened," and he said that, in that moment, he felt more happiness than he had ever felt in his life—ever! As it turned out, this came to the attention of the prison authorities. They reviewed his case, and, considering the age at which he had made his mistake in breaking the law, his sentence was reduced, and he was eventually released.

When interviewed later in his life he said, "It was a hell of a way to 'Wake Up,' but I'm so grateful for it. If I had gone on with my life without this experience I might likely would have never Awakened—and even more likely, would now be dead." It's a moving story and a deep lesson for all of us.

LETTING GO OF THE OLD AND REINVENTING YOURSELF

This is why I love Yoga so much. I have had wonderful mentors who helped me to understand "that something had changed" and could provide really wise and skillful feedback about how my path was progressing.

Whether it is weight you are carrying on your body, or some other attribute you take as plaguing your self-image, you can actually learn to let go of that self-image. You can make a change—dress in white, representing the purity of the practice, and show you are a woman who walks with nobility and grace. That may be the best you can at the stage you are in, but it's an important step. You can learn how to put a coil of hair on top of your head, tucking it under a covering, and believe it will actually hold your solar energies inside of you. When you see how people are drawn to you, you will know it's not just because you have fabulous hair but because your aura, your vibration, is saying something that moves them. You're trying; you're changing. And if the most you're achieving is just a good night's sleep, that is a gauge itself.

The Great Masters call that a "lever." In your Yogic life, you will find your life becomes full of levers, and each one is a gauge. How am I? Am I sleeping well, or do I go to bed with lots of chaos in my head? Does it take me hours to fall asleep? Do I have energy to clean my own house? Do I have energy to make my own food, or do I always have to order out?

You can see Yoga working. That is one of the most fulfilling parts of the adventure. You see your habits changing, changing into habits that feel good and make you feel happy—happy about yourself. That is what takes you to every new level of your maturity, even

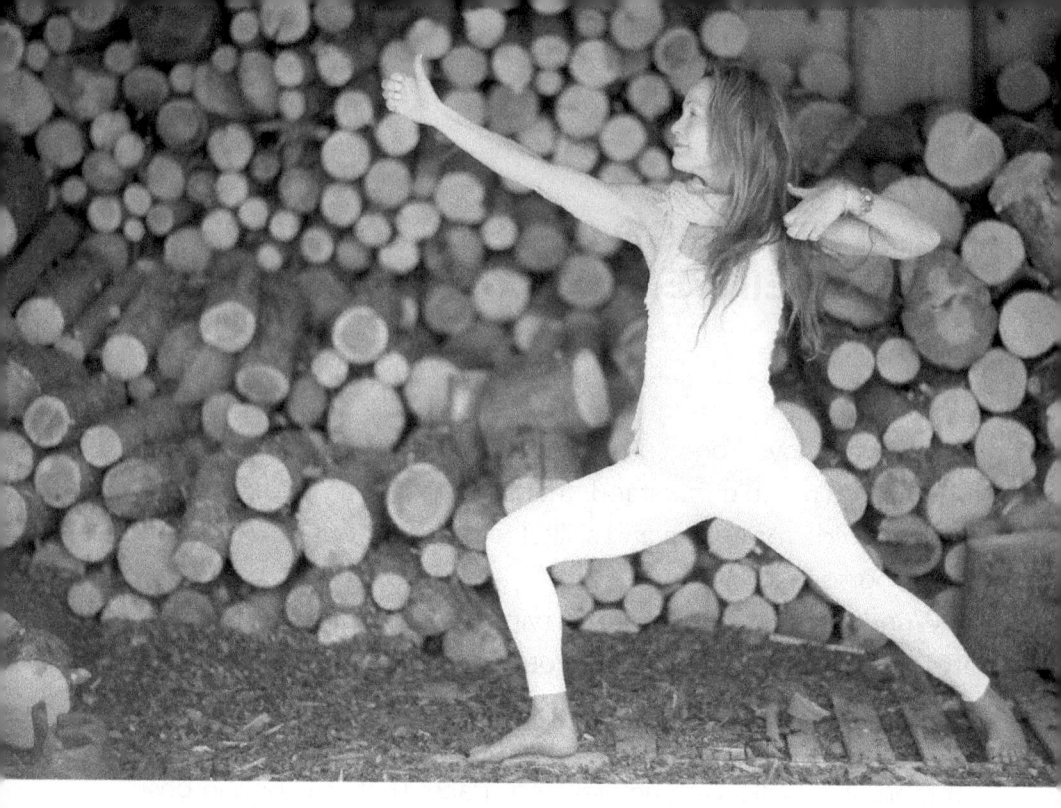

Bullseye

without any conventional benchmarks like diplomas, certificates, or degrees.

Measuring the Steps

How do we measure our steps of "Growing Up" within our "Waking Up?"

Well, for sure, in our Growing Up, we can get caught in the "Cleaning Up"—because there may be so much of it to do. This is why it's so important that we keep exploring and probing within our practice. After all, we are dropping an old personality and old sets of habits. We are learning to trust that our "new way of being and doing"—discovered in our practice—can replace our old one, completely. But we will naturally have some hesitancy in stepping more and more fully into this "new me." I don't know anyone who ever "woke up" who at some point didn't ask, "Can this new world

I've discovered *really cover* every aspect of the old one?" When you find that it can, and does so even better, it's a big step.

These transitions are even more difficult, however, if we have already had one, two, or even more career identities (even successful ones). We are bringing them all into this transition, and each has piled up a lot of files in our psychic and emotional system. I know what that's like. I was an over accomplisher, perhaps because I was raised in a sports-related competitive family. By the time I found Kundalini Yoga, I had two successful careers under my belt along with being a wife and mother. And because—having been in the major modeling business—I also had to change living locations and homes several times, I had to really learn to trust that there was an overriding Source that was leading all this.

I did have the advantage that in the modeling and acting business nothing is ever for sure, even if you are at the top. So, I was used to that. I knew the landscape of exploitive careers, no matter how lucrative, where everything depended on what you looked like, and who liked you, and whether you got a "break." But the twists and turns of my own unfolding comprised a still rather bizarre adventure—a rabbit hole for sure.

My Rabbit Hole and My Way Out

Here is how Source works sometimes. When I moved from working in Paris back to New York City, at age 21-22, I moved into an apartment, not only alone, but right near the Integral Yoga Center. I had already, much earlier—even without any exposure to Yoga—became a vegetarian. The real reason was I simply didn't like "regular food." So, I had basically changed my way of eating and became a vegetarian without any guidance and without any connection to spirituality. It was all very odd actually, which is sometimes how these things work. I had always been both athletic *and* deeply connected to nature—and I had long had this wonderful memory of how eating wheatgrass at age 16 had made me feel so wonderful.

This was a deeply ingrained pattern of my being able to listen to myself that had been going on for some time. Even when I went to Paris to model, it had unfolded in that extremely personalized way. Someone saw me and sent me to an agent, oddly enough named The Light Company. For some reason, I was courageous and self-assured enough to simply accept a one-way ticket to Paris into a world that was obviously beckoning me but about which I knew really nothing. Who gave me that courage? Why did I do that? So, there is a truth, I think, about subtle self-knowledge and how it leads us to these points of Awakening, different points of Awakening, all the time.

So, you get to your twenties and you're "a player," making a lot of money, going to all the fancy nightclubs, dancing all night, and, all the while, also meeting amazing photographers and representatives. Then somehow, you reach about age 25, and you suddenly start to wake up to a mixed landscape. Some things, so satisfying before, are not so satisfying. Somehow, all the pictures they are taking of you don't seem like you anymore. What felt like achievement yesterday starts feeling a bit like old news. You start to feel, somehow deeply, that something else must be up ahead.

This is challenging because, as you enter this kind of twist and turn, you are often on your own. You realize: "Oh, they don't want to hear about me. They aren't interested in my real life. They just want to *see* me." So, luckily, I then married and moved to London, and a whole new vista opened—the chance to attend the Bristol Old Vic Theatre School. Here, they didn't care at all what I looked like. It's what I had to *say* that interested them.

My Next Chapter

For me, this next unfolding chapter was equally odd, and in a very personalized way. My move to London and now being married to a very successful, and conservative, British businessman set up a perhaps inevitable collision between conventional priorities of that life and my desire to also make good of new possibilities. With equal intensity of attending to my family responsibilities, I set my sights on applying to the Bristol Old Vic Theatre School. Perhaps the most celebrated school of its kind in Britain, it schools not only actors but also every niche of the theatre trade for film, radio, and TV as well. It lists over forty famous alumni—Daniel Day Lewis, Sophie Thompson, Jeremy Irons, Miranda Richardson, Gene Wilder, Patrick Stewart, and Olivia Colman, to just name a few. Perhaps I was lucky that my initial intents were not taken all that seriously by those around me.

But when I got a callback from my audition, things stirred quickly. My callback itself is a funny story. I was asked to recite a monologue in some unique way. So, what did I do? I stood on my head and recited the monologue! For some reason, that's what I was drawn to do. I had always enjoyed playing, and this just seemed to be the thing to do. Why not? My callback must have been compelling, as I was accepted into the Bristol Old Vic Theatre School. I was, by then, also the mother of two small children, with a very loving husband.

So, I would please everyone. I would get up at 4:30 AM, put dinner in the oven for that night, then put breakfast on the table, and head out for school. I did that every single day until I graduated from Theatre School. There was never ever a feeling that I was a great actress, and to be honest, it was a complete and utter struggle. As well, my self-confidence was not buffered with a lot of encouragement from others. I had to be my own best encouragement. But there was some kind of drive, some determination, in me that would not go away.

This was an Awakening in itself because I had cleared away so much stuff by then. Before I auditioned for the Old Vic, I had also become a helicopter pilot. That probably surprises you, but my husband was a pilot. When I flew with him it would occur to me, "What if he had a heart attack? I would need to take over." I became one of fourteen women in Britain at the time with a helicopter license.

Again, oddly, as Source would have it, I'll never forget my flight instructor. He became a big fan of mine and was constantly encouraging me about everything I wanted to do. That was rare and welcome! He made me realize that I had some special gifts that I wasn't being encouraged to use. He constantly encouraged me in that little Bell 47 to believe I could do anything I wanted. He even set me up for my first solo flight by simply jumping out of the plane. He had that much confidence in me. Even to this day, I remember him when I am encouraging students and really urging them to probe into the unknown and to test their limits.

So, in the journey, it's not what you're doing but how you are doing it. It's taking a risk–with your marriage, with your children, with yourself. But everything can change when you truly find yourself. So, I stuck with everything. I got the lead role in *Bartholomew Fair*, the famous Jacobean comedy by Ben Jonson. It was perfect for me, and we had a good run. But what I remember most is my children sitting in the balcony watching their mother perform–and my being amused when my son's only comment was (since I had to drink beer in the part), "Mom you don't drink beer!"

I guess you could say everything in my life has been about waking up. And I'm very thankful and blessed that I could make the mistakes I did in my life and still be not only OK with them, but also acknowledge them as stepping stones toward others and their Awakening and toward a deep understanding of community, forgiveness, and friendship. I learned we never have to be afraid about reinventing ourselves. Often, it is a part of our destiny.

RADICALLY BEING YOU

You've heard the adages "Be yourself, everyone is taken!" and "Be yourself, the rest of the universe will adjust!" or this line from an old song "I love you just the way you are." There is a Great Teacher who says, "Be yourself–*radically*! Love who and what you love, and simply try to do your best by them all."

When is it that you give yourself that permission to take the bull by the horns and say to yourself, "I am what I am. You can kick me out or you can keep me, love me or not, because I trust where I'm delivering my practice, understanding, and teaching. My practice is exactly where I need to be."

We are all unique, and it's important to study the radical edges on who we each are. And, you can explore all these radical edges without doing yourself or anyone else any harm. Some Great Teachers call this "discovering your own ground," your own "bottom line," or "standing in your Awareness" on that ground. You are not replaceable; you are a distinct vessel whose permutations can only come from what you uniquely are. Sometimes, this is the "four eyes" conversation you have just between you and God.

Think about Stephen Hawking for a moment–the great astrophysicist and cosmologist who, completely crippled just at the time of his emerging genius in early university, could not walk or use his hands and, eventually, could only speak through a computer. He was not perfect. He made mistakes. His relationships with loved ones were not always a model, but through this unique person was revealed some of the most important theories and understandings of modern science.

Think of the athletes who created the Special Olympics because their spirit wanted to show that no amount of disability or challenge could keep them from experiencing and sharing the competitive spirit of sports. Some of the greatest discoveries of, and gifts to, humankind were from those who explored totally new frontiers.

Davy Crockett, the great American pioneer who died defending the Alamo, is famous for saying, "Be sure you're right. Then go ahead." A two-time Congressman from Kentucky, he is the only Congressman in history to have not been able to read or write. But, a fiery orator, known for his integrity and honesty, he was a champion for both the environment and for indigenous peoples. The destructive elements of the American government at that time spent the equivalent of millions of dollars to have him defeated and removed from Congress. He died at the Alamo with other Americans who felt that America had become so corrupt that they needed a new start—the Republic of Texas. We don't remember the names of those who persecuted him, but Crockett is famous.

If someone else thinks you're replaceable, that's *their* story, and, as we mature, we all learn not to get caught in other people's stories. As one great philosopher said, "Be sure to know whose problems are whose." This can help you to be sure of yourself and to have the courage to explore the frontiers that are a part of your own destiny.

There is much to be said of the person who has discovered who they are and, giving themselves permission, then decides the story they will create for *their* story, in this lifetime. As the spiritual teacher Robert Adams (who reported he had lived with Ramana Maharshi much of his life) said, "When you have cleaned your house, then you can decide who your guests are." This is a proud moment, deep inside. When we realize that our stories are not necessarily who we are, we learn we can, and also must, choose our stories carefully.

In this time, we have the opportunity to choose many stories for ourselves, to wear many hats—even simultaneously—and it's important that we do. As my Denver friend, philosopher Ken Wilber says, we live at a time when all the wisdom resources of the world are on the table—at our beck and call through modern media, especially the internet. The COVID-era taught us we can have conversations with friends around the world 24-7, as often as we like. It's a time in history when we could, all together, make the turn to serve the whole world.

Ken Wilber is himself an example of radically being himself and building the story he chose. Today, he is considered to be "the Einstein of Consciousness," a role that was seized through his own surety about his life and destiny. Seeking a "philosophy of everything," he dropped out of the conventional track of graduate schools to take "the express train" based on his own sense of direction. Soon, the world will be celebrating (actually!) a fifth decade anniversary of the publication of Wilber's seminal book *The Spectrum of Consciousness* (January 1, 1977). At the time of its original publication, it had been rejected by more than twenty publishers; it was that far ahead of its time. Today, over twenty books later, in twenty-five languages, he is acknowledged as a trailblazing integral philosopher, leaving in the dust those who said he should have been less bold, and waiting out the long, often twisted and incorrect, processes of professional publishing "peer review." Ramana Maharshi once said that, in such situations, such titans of self-knowledge often simply find innocent dogs yapping at their heels, unable to understand what it means to pave your own way. Wilber, of course, has written eloquently about this struggle in his book *Grace and Grit*.

This is not to say that every exercise in senses of self-destiny is always of the sacred variety, and this is a lesson in itself. We know there are examples of skewed, twisted versions of such self-assurance, and they are a part of what we also learn in recognizing the sacred from the profane or delusional. Adolf Hitler's secretary reported that when he decided to invade Russia and ignore what had happened to everyone who had tried before—like Napoleon—Hitler shook his fist at the sky and dared the gods to try and stop him. We've seen what can happen when self-assurance takes a delusional, or simply evil, turn.

If our species does not master this precipice—of what can drive human ego—we likely will never see the world based on the Heart of which so many of us dream. As His Holiness the 14th Dalai Lama recently summarized in a discussion with my friend Dr. Kurt Johnson, "The problem is this: in today's world, the high values are most often not where the tractions of power are, and the tractions of power are most often not where the high values are." When we understand the moral and ethical differences between the world of the heart we want to see and so many landscapes of human pathology and suffering today, we can clearly see what is at stake.

It is one thing to choose stories for ourselves; this is something common to all. It is quite another when we start to take responsibility for our communities and, even beyond that, for our planet. We are at a turning point for this beloved planet of ours. We honestly do not have that much time to put straight everything that is out of line in our world.

As many of you know, I am also an adopted pipe carrier in one of the Sioux Nation traditions, where I am also ordained as a "Wisdom Keeper." My name in that tradition is *Chanté Eton Wo Wa Gla Ka Win*, which means "Woman that Speaks from the Heart." I'll say much more about Mother Earth, Mother Gaia, and our responsibility to Her at the end of this book.

These are parts of the many faces of Karuna, in my world of "Radically Be Yourself": Carrie, Caroline, Livpreet Kaur, Karuna, Rev. Karuna. The story, the journey, continues. The many names met me along the unknown of walking my path. They were exactly right for where I was in my life at the time, and each was a step of the Way.

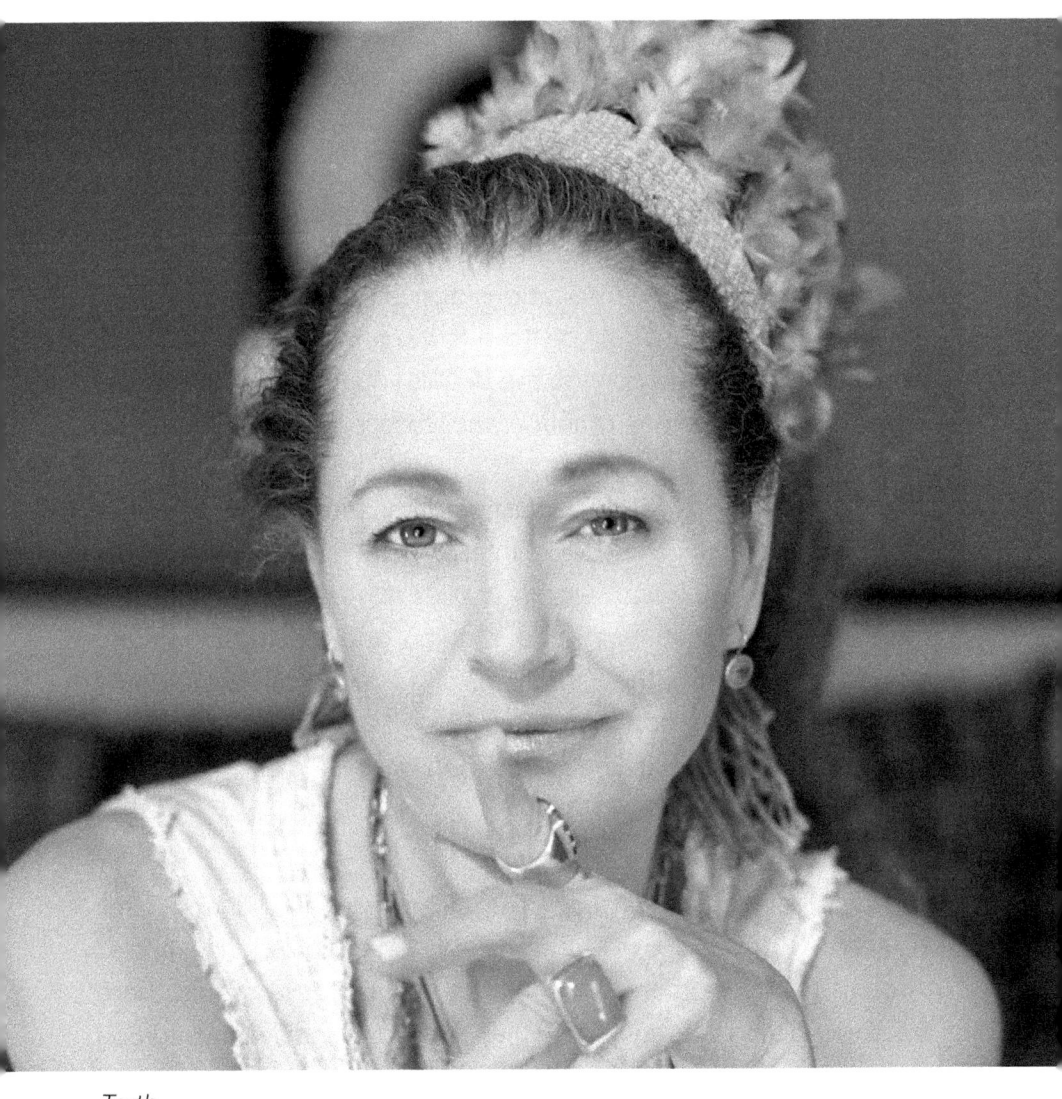

Truth

LIFESTYLE

FINDING OUR SPIRITUAL PRACTICE

Yoga

I've spoken about Yoga already many times in this book. In fact, I have used the word over 600 times. You know, it is my practice and my path. All of my inspirations above have pointed to Yoga, and I said, in introducing you to this book, we would start with inspirations and then move to the details you need to know about Yoga history, cosmology, practice, and lifestyle. So, regarding those, let's now take a deep look.

The landscape of "Yoga" is vast, and it is the subject of tens of thousands of books worldwide. Interestingly, historians and other scholars apply multiple meanings even to the word itself. It is generally agreed that Yoga is about "union" and specifically "uniting human spirit" with "the Divine." But its technical "etymology" (word origins) is far more rich and nuanced–as I explained in detail previously in "What Has Led You to Finding This Book."

History of Yoga

Yoga's chronological history is equally enigmatic, dating back at least 5,000 years, 3,000 before our current calendar era, and through the more than 2,000 years since. Because of this, there are Yogic histories in multiple cultures. Because my root tradition in Yoga is Kundalini Yoga and, more specifically, in the Sikh tradition, even though I will share much more about the historical landscape of Yoga worldwide, much of what I share of techniques and methods will be from my root tradition.

Given the universality of Yoga, many of the practices and techniques have companions across the other traditions. This in itself makes them universally useful but, further, serves the specific purpose of sharing practices *that are known to work* in these great traditions.

Even in my further comments below, on Yogic history and philosophy, I'll speak from the Sikh "entry point" on Yogic history, which paints the panorama much as below.

History sees Yogic practice extending across the entire landscape of Hinduism (a very broad term in itself), Buddhism, Jainism, and Sikhism, to use only a few convenient categories. Sikhism comes on the scene in the 15th and 16th Century. The history of its primal founder, Guru Nanak (1469-1539), and of its foundational scriptures, the *Guru Granth Sahib*, are rich not only in a multifaith heritage from across the Old World at that time, but also in discussions of the heritage and practices of Yoga.

Guru Nanak himself propounded a "Sahaja" or "Nama" Yoga centering on "meditation" on the Name. But, later, Sikh practitioners revisited the Yogic heritage of the roots of the Sikh tradition and led a renaissance in the practices and techniques that are now associated with Kundalini Yoga. That is my root tradition and also one in which international interfaith organizations have ordained me as a "Wisdom Keeper." Because I am privileged to be the Host Editor of *Light on Light Magazine* (which annually does a Special Issue with the United Nations Committee for the International Day of Yoga), I see—every year—the panorama of Yogic practice across the world roll out in front of my eyes.

To be more specific then, about the history of Yoga, the Sikh lens sees nine great "Epochs" of Yoga.

The Prehistoric Period (from before 2000 BCE)
There are no historical writings *per se* from this period but there are numerous cultural accounts that point to the development of spiritual, meditational, and physical techniques for spiritual development, health, and well-being.

The Vedic Period (2000-1000 BCE)
With the writings of the Mahabharata on the Indian subcontinent and the mixing of subcultures and races across even a larger Eurasian region, Yogic practice became a cultural axis. Foundational writings and scripture fundamental to Yoga appear from this period—the "Books of Knowledge" like the Rig-Veda, the Sama-Veda, the Yajur-Veda, and the Atharva-Veda. Music also became a primary vehicle for spiritual practice and observance.

The Brahmanic Period (1000-800 BCE)
Yogic practice became formalized and ritualistic and, with a hierarchy of leadership, less supportive of the essence and mystical elements of the traditions. Yogic practice became more formally religious and less spiritual.

The Upanishadic Period (800-500 BCE)
There is a renaissance of the spiritual foundations of Yoga particularly through the Upanishad writings [*Upanishad* itself meaning to "be mystically near" the Source]. It is an era of great gurus and great teachers and innovative and creative new horizons for Yogic techniques for realization and transformation. Raj Yoga and Kundalini Yoga, emphasizing "direct path" and "natural awakened awareness," became rich traditions.

The Gita Period (500 BCE- 200 CE)
The richness of the former period synergized into great works of spiritual writings, like the Ramayana (an epic poem) and the Bhagavad Gita (a dialogue between Krishna and his devotee, Prince Arjuna) which becomes part of the Mahabharata. These works portray classic archetypes of the human spiritual journey and our global evolution and became major parts of the global landscape of greatly influential spiritual works.

The Classical Period (200-800 CE)
This period is famous for the appearance of Patanjali's classic Yoga Sutras, wherein, during this time, the major schools of Yoga and Yogic philosophy (the "six schools") were systematized.

The Puranic Period (800-1470 CE)
Vedantic nondual mysticism matured during this period with the writing of "The Puranas" and the mystical teaching of Shankara. Central to many of the aspects of the "nonduality" of Vedanta was Yoga and Yogic techniques. Understanding of the chakras and aura and the discipline of Sadhana became prominent.

The Bhakti Period (1470-1710 CE)
Yogic practice mainstreamed across all walks of life with a melding of the traditions of devotion (Bhakti emphasis), the Guru (Sant emphasis), and Yoga's psycho-physical aspects (Tantric emphasis). During this period in the Sikh tradition produced The Ten Gurus and its great work of scripture: the *Siri Guru Granth Sahib*.

The Modern Period (1710 CE-present)
The history of Yoga became profoundly affected by the replacement of Moghul-Persian-Islamic rule across the Indian

sub-continent by British colonialism. Western influences included secularization and control of industry and labor by the foreign western powers. But a favorable outcome of this situation was the meeting of Eastern and Western spirituality and the gradual but persistent dissemination of Eastern spirituality, including Yoga, westward and throughout the world. The emerging post World War II global civilization saw a profound surge in global interest, popularity, and study of Eastern spirituality and Yoga.

This transformation, in which America played such an important role, is recorded panoramically in the well-known book by our colleague Philip Goldberg, *American Veda*.

As Goldberg shows, by the 20th Century, America became the center of global culture. And, growing outward from America's influence on the global culture were writers, philosophers, artists, and musicians bringing, knowingly or unknowingly, the profound insights of Eastern spirituality, including Yoga. Goldberg's subtitle says it well: "From Emerson and the Beatles to Yoga and Meditation How Indian Spirituality Changed the West."

East and West came together too. After the first Parliament of the World's Religions in 1893, India's famed Swami Vivekananda toured the world. Swami Yogananda's *Autobiography of a Yogi* was read by millions and was echoed by the mid-20th Century in the world's most popular literature and music—from J. D. Salinger's *Catcher in the Rye* and Hermann Hesse's *Siddhartha* and *Steppenwolf* to the music of the Beatles and every other musical group of that Eastern-influenced "psychedelic" era. It was a wild ride, but it brought the potentials of global wisdom together from East, West, North, and South.

It was in this era, as well, that the mysteries of Kundalini Yoga came westward from the Sikh tradition of India, particularly through the spiritual teacher Yogi Bhajan. Coming initially to Canada in 1968, he reached out to countless persons of that "60s" era who were struggling for new senses of identity and meaning. He became a well-known personage of the raucous "60s Guru Era"—with all its foibles. Some aspects of his character as a Yogi of that era are still controversial today—part of the age-old matter of the "Message and the Messenger." But, by the 21st Century, Kundalini Yoga had joined the twenty-some brands and flavors of Yogic practice as a mainstay of global Yogic heritage and practice.

Kundalini Yoga distinguishes itself from some other forms of Yoga by its emphasis on the more deeply spiritual, meditational, and subtle-realm elements of Yogic practice. Although, yes, it utilizes all the poses and postures ("asanas," "mudras," "kriyas," etc.) and other actions today familiar across our world's commercialization of Yoga, these are more deeply rooted in the Ancient Wisdom in Kundalini Yoga and, thus, embodied with more creativity, variety, and flexibility—and *yet* with great precision.

Thus, Kundalini Yoga is often acknowledged as a "deeper dive" into the vast landscape of Yoga, distinguishing it in many ways from the commercial Yogas that have often become just another exercise form or "day in the gym." Because Kundalini Yoga so deeply links to authentic spirituality, this is why many practitioners of the other, more commercial, Yogas clamor to it once they have tasted its rare and amazing gifts.

It is uniquely anchored in both the Wisdom of the world's Great Spiritual Traditions as well as our modern-day understandings of Consciousness and "nonduality"—authentic Awakening—especially as it relates to the activity of our body's "Kundalini energy."

So, welcome to this amazing landscape!

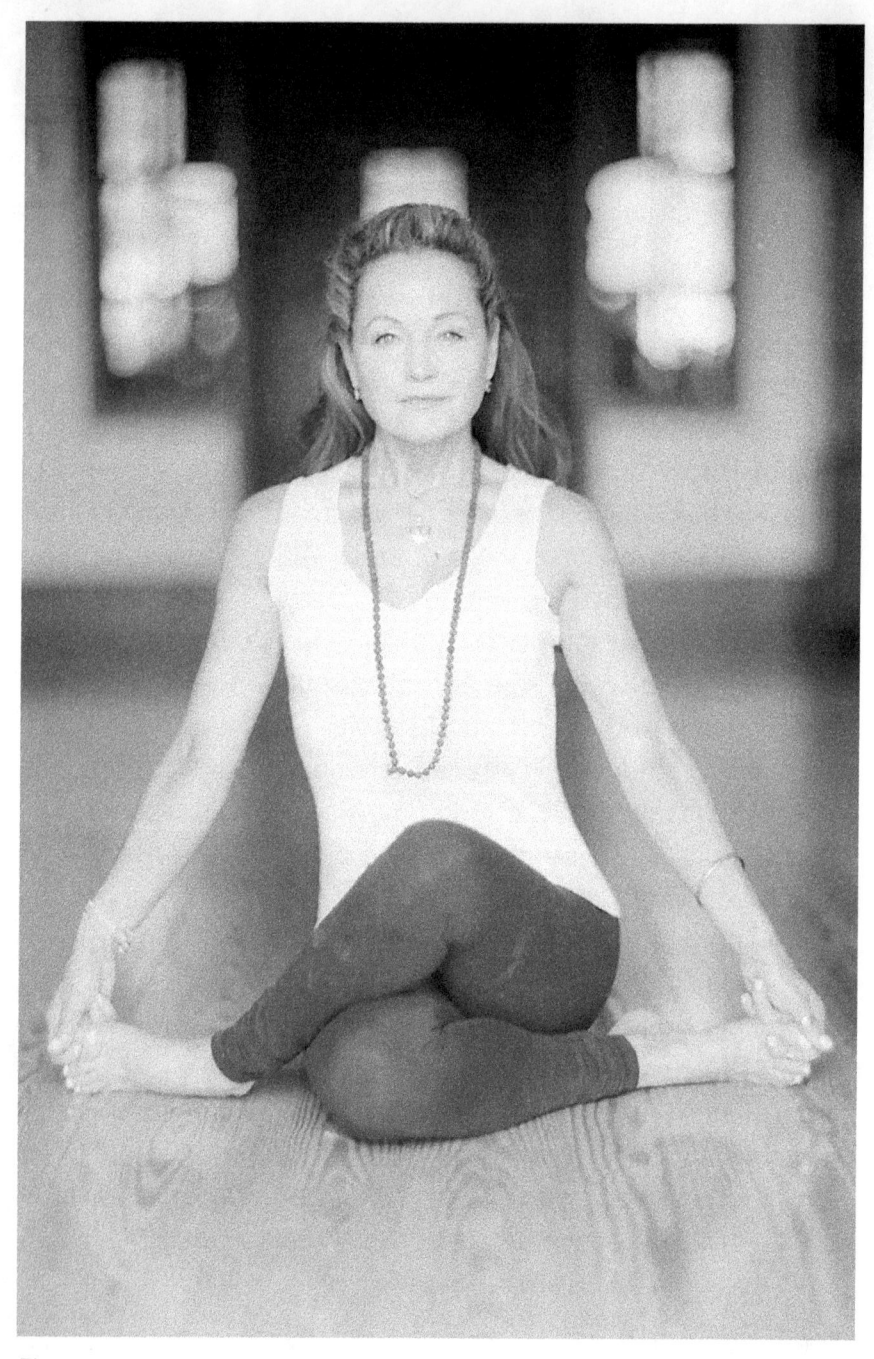

Eloquence

Distinguishing Kundalini Yoga

Drawing from multi-faith roots, Kundalini Yoga is distinctive in its emphasis on the deeply mystical and subtle-realm knowledge that underpins all of Yoga's worldwide heritage. While it employs the myriad poses and postures ("asanas," "mudras," "kriyas," etc.) familiar from today's popular Yoga, it anchors profoundly in ancient Yoga cosmology and its finely nuanced understanding of the Awakening process. This puts it also in stride with our modern neuroscientific understandings of "nondual consciousness" and the role of the body in nurturing the highest potential for authentic Awakening and actualizing our fullest moral and ethical capacity. In a vision of a world Waking Up and Growing Up, such an emphasis is paramount. Let's look now at the entire landscape we need to understand with regard to Yoga practice.

Elements of the Kundalini Yoga Landscape

Kundalini Yoga activity typically involves these intertwined elements. Each is fully elaborated herein in the Yoga Practice Appendices specially assembled for the practices chosen for this book. These are drawn from my larger comprehensive Yoga Manual–[*The Light on Kundalini Yoga Manual*]–a 2024 e-publication from my Light on Kundalini community (see https://lightonkundalini.com/).

The Manual is structured the same way Yoga practices are organized in this book–as *"Foundational," "Day to Day,"* and *"Sessional."* As well, many sessions also appear in *Light on Light Magazine* and my online courses at Sacred U and and on Humanity's Stream,

- https://issuu.com/lightonlight
- https://courses.sacredstories.com/
- https://stream.humanitysteam.org/awakening-the-ten-bodies-with-karuna

- https://stream.humanitysteam.org/healing-grief-with-karuna
- https://stream.humanitysteam.org/3-minute-meditations-with-karuna
- https://stream.humanitysteam.org/81-facets-of-mind-with-karuna)

and you will be guided to these as well. These elements are:

- "Mantras"–that is, "chants"
- "Prayers"–that is, traditional prayer, but especially from the ancient Wisdom Traditions
- "Mudras"–that is, positions of the hands and fingers
- "Drishti"–that is, considerations of focus or gaze
- "Bandhas"–that is, "locks" of the body's various muscles for specific purposes of guiding energy
- "Breath Work" (or "Pranayama")–that is, breath-related attention and exercises
- "Asanas"–that is, various of the traditional "postures" of Yoga
- "Meditation"–that is, immersion in silence or guided consciousness exercises"
- "Kriyas"–that is, prescribed sequences of all the above

So, now let's look at some of the basic elements you will need to have familiarity with to continue your journey into this amazing Yogic landscape.

The Chakras

Before moving on to understanding more of the philosophy and cosmology of Yoga, you will want to be acquainted with the Chakras. They are fundamental to all Yogic understanding both in the formless world of the spiritual and the material world of form. In fact, often they are seen as the interface between these two companion dimensions.

In the Yogic traditions, Kundalini (in Sanskrit meaning "coiled snake") is the primordial cosmic energy lying at the base of the spine and, in metaphor, then ascends through the chakras as a part of spiritual "awakening." The possibility of this awakening is seen as the birthright of every person.

Understanding the Chakras is a heritage shared by all the great traditions, although there is some variance in how this is detailed. Consistent with the general concepts of contemporary Yoga, which are drawn from the millennial Vedic traditions of the Indian subcontinent, the Chakras are generally portrayed as below. They are seen as seven centers (hubs, loci, or interfaces) located along the spine and associated with multiple physiological functions and also spiritual implications that are physical, emotional, and mental.

Here are the Chakras listed in ascending order, including the name in English common usage, their Sanskrit name, the general locations, and the color assigned to the Chakra by the mystical traditions.

1. Root Chakra ("*Muladhara*")–base of the spine–red
2. Sacral Chakra ("*Svadhisthana*")–just below the navel–orange
3. Solar Plexus Chakra ("*Manipura*")–stomach area–yellow
4. Heart Chakra ("*Anahata*")–center of the chest–green
5. Throat Chakra ("*Vishuddha*")–base of the throat–blue
6. Third Eye Chakra("*Ajna*")–forehead, above between the eyes–indigo
7. Crown Chakra ("*Sahasrara*")–top of the head–violet

This knowledge of the Chakras allows a basic understanding of the Bandhas (Locks) about which more detail is provided in the Foundational Yoga Practice Appendix 1 in this book and in my Yoga Manual. The Bandhas (Locks) are applied through the muscles around certain areas of the spine to align the body for energy transfer and also to prevent misaligned energy movement.

In this way, the action resembles "locks" in a dam which align the movement of water. In actual Yoga practice, however, because the Bandhas (Locks) are applied as a constriction with some finesse, not with undue force, they are sometimes described as more gentle, even flower-like, openings and closings (constrictions and relaxations) to direct energy along the spine. In general, the locks are applied while holding, or as part of, a posture and most often as directed by the Teacher.

Yoga Cosmology

Yoga cosmology—Yoga's view of Source, the universe, and everything in it—comes from thousands of years of observing patterns and inter-relationships, from the time of the ancients until now. Its view of life unfolds throughout the Vedic texts—the writings of the great spiritual traditions of the Indian subcontinent. It is a cosmology in which everything is interconnected, from the smallest to the largest, from the worlds of galaxies and solar systems to the daily lives of human beings. The wisdom in it, tested over and over by time, embraces all aspects of human life—the spirit, the mind, the body, and all the interconnected elements needed for our health and well-being.

Since the soul, mind, and body are all connected to how this cosmology works, it is in that context that we can claim a birthright to the most meaningful and healthy of lives. Undoubtedly, this is why Yoga, now also tested out in the West in recent centuries, has achieved its great popularity—mostly simply, because it works.

The cosmology of Yoga, the narratives of its ancient spiritual texts, and its view of the oneness of the human body with the entire design of the universe are all intimately interconnected. They interconnect soul, body, and mind with the minutest of details of lifestyle—moving from the great overall wisdoms to all the minute details of diet and health, as in the revered traditions of Ayurveda (about which I will provide a separate section). It is all one comprehensive cosmology.

Living as we do in the 21st Century, looking back some 5,000 years since the origins of these Yogic views, we now have the chance of exploring and employing any, or all, of this vast array of offerings from this amazing heritage.

Yoga and the Structure of Everything

It is important for us to realize and remember when we are participating in Yoga across any of its more than twenty schools or varieties today—not to mention the context of its vast popularity today—that its roots are ancient. Yes, you could participate in the most superficial, exercise-related activities of Yoga and reap their benefits without referencing this rich ancient heritage. But you would not be able to access the depths of its gifts—especially the possibility of true conscious Awakening and the riches of its knowledge of health and well-being—without some understanding of its worldview, its cosmology. This is because everything in the minutest detail regarding Yoga—the understanding of how Yoga works, why it works, and the connection of that to its wisdoms regarding health, diet, fitness, and well-being—all flows from its comprehensive view of the universe and you.

So, let's connect you to a basic understanding of the worldview—the cosmology—of Yoga. For that, we'll use a metaphor, or comparison, that, although not perfect, works very well. An easy way to comprehend Yoga cosmology's way of connecting the largest and the smallest is to think of the relationship of sunlight falling on your face, and the Sun from which the light is emanating. Science calls the elements that make up light "photons." So, sunlight is photons streaming from the Sun. *And,* the Sun itself is a gigantic cluster of photons. But, we obviously recognize that the light experienced on our faces is not the Sun itself, nor is the Sun itself the same as the light on our face. They are parts of a continuum but have their own unique identities. It should not surprise us then that the metaphor is also true at the minutest level. Photons themselves are mysterious entities (called "quanta" by science) that are waves *and* particles at the same time.

This is a useful metaphor about how the cosmology of Yoga understands the intimate connection between ourselves and "the Divine" and, thus, ascribes to us the "birthright" of being able to attain an awakened life of happiness and well-being. Using the metaphor of the relationship of light and the Sun we can understand the Yogic vision of how these realms are interconnected. The landscape, or map, of that interconnection in all its details explains the whole of life as comprehended in Yogic cosmology. This landscape is portrayed below because all the elements of Yoga, from the worldview of Yoga to Yoga practice and Yoga lifestyle (like Ayurveda), are all one cosmology.

In this cosmology, all of Nature—like all the light from the Sun, the Sun, and the light shining on your face—is called, together, in Sanskrit, *Prakriti*. As the *all* of Nature, it includes everything both material and immaterial—what is in form and what is formless—everything. That which is still formless, called *Parusha*, is like the light streaming from the Sun—that is, from Source (*Shiva*)—to its "becoming" in the diverse world of active multiplicity (*Shakti*), some thing, or energy, in the world of form. Source is, in that sense, always "manifesting." As it plays in the manifest world, it is alive in the realm of our human senses. Here, obviously it is in play with all that humans experience and embody, the whole spectrum from confusion to clarity. This multiplicity of forms and activities and how we humans comprehend them is called *Maya*—the predicament in which humans find themselves.

Yoga and Our Human Predicament (Gunas)

In this predicament, of our human life in real time, Yoga recognizes major elements of how humans comprehend things–the *"Gunas"*–the spectrum of conditions of matter and mind. Three are generalized–three because they recognize two extremes and that which joins them. These *Gunas*, senses or lens, are *Sattva*, which is when we can see clearly and know what is actually true; *Tamas*, which we see things confused and uncertain; and *Rajas*, when sense is willful, and energetic, moving with the intention to clarify and find out what is true.

Of course, the three qualities are always intertwined in our world of experience, always interacting with each other and in flux.

The interactions of the three Gunas make up *"Chitta"*–the world of the mind. In *Chitta*, the Gunas manifest in a reflected array:

Tamas–the basic sense of sensory mind, our raw senses of things (external sounds, and images, but also the internal ones of feelings, even subconscious reactions);

Sattva–the Awakened (*Buddhi*) mind, which comprehends clearly, discerns well, and sees what it true, even in the largest infinite senses; and

Rajas–as *"Ahangkar"* (the ego sense), in which we experience a sense of identity, sense of self, and "who we are versus 'others'."

As we all know, our world of the mind–*Chitta*–is always a mixture of all of these. In our lives, they all intermix across our sense of emotion, our sensory input and output, and our experience of the material world–our sense of being substantial, of "being here" with other material things. Across all of these, of course, we also experience limits and boundaries, restrictions which limit and confine power, knowledge, desire, time, space, and so on.

It is from this complexity, which we all experience, that the intricacies of our tendencies, potentialities, and their dynamics of flux exist in both our conscious and subconscious minds. These are, in Yoga cosmology, the "*Samskaras*" of our lives, the very rabbit hole we started with in this book. It is this complex and confusing experience of life to which Yoga brings its skills—the "This Way Out" I championed in OUR JOURNEY in this book.

The *samskaras*, or the jungle created by all of our sensory worlds, have myriad causes and interacting elements, of course. They comprise "who we are" as biological organisms, where the foibles of our brains and nervous systems either work well—or don't. Involved are our entire encyclopedias of experience, memories—all the content we have—which I will explain to you much more later as "the *Akasha*" or "Akashic Record." In our minds and emotions, these all play through our myriads of likes and dislikes, thoughts and impulses, and what motivates us to action, be they helpful or harmful. They manifest as all the dimensions of psychology and psychiatry. Given all this complexity, the Yoga cosmology of the Sikh tradition, from which comes most of the heritage of Kundalini Yoga, recognizes 9 aspects, 27 projections, and 81 facets of the mind. I'll say that again: 9 aspects, 27 projections, and 81 facets of the mind.

But what is important is not this minute analysis, but the more universal understanding of what actions we can take as human beings—what practices we can take up and master, as in Yogic practice—to find that birthright and destiny that is ours, a happy life of deepest well-being.

Yoga and Finding the Birthright

The way out of the rabbit hole, the path to a good life, lies in the realm of understanding the Divine aspects inherent in our consciousness.

These include the role of will, intention, choice, and volition—and—how these relate to the "limbs"—the elements—of Yoga available to us as "our way out." In the jungle of the *samskaras,* we discover that we have clear and distinctive viewpoints for our navigation within the confusions and challenges of that jungle. Yoga calls these lenses deep within us the "three minds." Yoga also understands that once these minds are utilized to their full capacity, the role of the will—of spiritual intention—is then fully energized, further honing our direction toward the birthright I speak of above.

The three minds are our thinking modes as positive, negative, and neutral. They act very clearly—just like "yes," "no," or "maybe"—and each has distinct assets.

The asset of our *positive mind* is its nature as expansive and embracing. It seeks positive results in creativity, fulfillment, and achievement; it is energetic and adventurous toward success.

The asset of our *negative mind* is that it is protective. Accordingly, it monitors threat, danger, or pain and pursues what will protect us.

The asset of *neutral mind* is that, locked in neither the emotions of negative or positive reaction, it is calm, measured, and non-attached, capable of acute discernment and strategic, well thought out actions.

All three minds are important to our maximum attainment of the skills and assets of Yogic practice, assisting each in achieving their fullest capacity. Among the classic Eight Limbs of Yoga, the Yoga postures (*asanas*) and breathwork (*pranayama*) aid in the development and full capacity of positive mind. The behavioral disciplines and ethical practices of Yoga (*yamas* and *niyamas*) do the same for negative mind, and the meditative practices—pratyahara (transcending the senses), *dharana* (concentrative meditation), *dhyana* (absorption practice), *samadhi* (states of union)—all enhance the serving skills of neutral mind.

These ancient understandings interestingly parallel modern neuroscience's knowledge of various evolutionary levels of our brain-mind that also attentively serve us. Our latent "reptilian brain" acts in fight-or-flight response to protect us. Our "mammalian" brain, the frontal cortex, provides higher analytical capacities for confident, creative thought and action. Advanced cortical capacities add the dimensions that we witness in highly spiritual people, manifesting exceptional clarity and discernment, and even spiritual gifts or powers (*siddhis*).

These skills of positive, negative, and neutral mind in Yogic practice are then applied with will and intention, understanding how—acting from either desire and emotion or clarity of mind—we can perform at highest capacity.

It is in these contexts of Yoga cosmology that Patanjali described the Eight Limbs of Yogic practice:

Asana—the postures of Yogic practice,
Pranayama—breathwork,
Yama—the disciplines of ethical living,
Niyama—the affirmation of highest ethics,
Pratyahara—the mastery of sense and thought,
Dhyana—the practices of meditation,
Dharana—the single-pointed power of intention, and
Samadhi—Awakening to enlightened consciousness.

It is the interrelation of these two domains—the elements of Yoga cosmology, and their relationship to Yogic health and well-being—that we will wrap together as this book continues. But let's start with Yoga practice itself.

Yoga Practice

Practicing Yoga is a developmental and evolutionary landscape that works from initial, foundational, understanding to more advanced understanding and practices, all of which build outward and upward—much like limbs and branches of a tree. It was with this metaphor that Patanjali penned the most famous historical work on Yoga—his 2nd Century *Yoga Sutras*—describing "The Eight Limbs of Yoga."

The most exciting and fulfilling part of your Yoga practice will be building it step by step and discovering what really works for you—and then building further and further. You will see the progress not only in your physical health and emotional and spiritual well-being, but also in new and expanding levels of discovery.

So, let's begin by introducing you to the foundational elements of Yoga practice—the rudimentary tools—that will be necessary for you to have in hand to begin this journey. Later, as the landscape and horizons in this book continue to augment and expand, I will spend much more time on each aspect. This will be true not only in what I further explain and elaborate but also when I provide specific Yoga practices for you to enhance your ever-growing experience of the Yogic journey and its inevitable destination in Awakening.

The Four Foundational Elements of Yoga – from Kundalini Yoga

The Foundational Elements include an understanding of the most basic elements of the Yogic landscape from which all the other members, or limbs, are built. The fundamental components are used and built from across the myriad varieties that comprise the totality of Yogic practice. So, I will include:

1. *Foundational Knowledge of Body Postures ("Asanas") and Hand and Finger Positions ("Mudras") that are either regularly employed, or which built-out from, in various varieties and combinations*
2. *Foundational Knowledge of the Breathwork ("Pranayama") and Mantra*

3. *Foundational Knowledge of the Bandhas ("Locks") and the Chakras*
4. *Foundational Knowledge of the Elements of Yoga Daily Practice ("Foundational," "Day to Day," and "Sessional")*

Below, I will introduce these one by one, from the order above. Later in the book, I will provide much more detail and elaboration, in the special section of "INSPIRED MESSAGES *with Yoga Practices."*

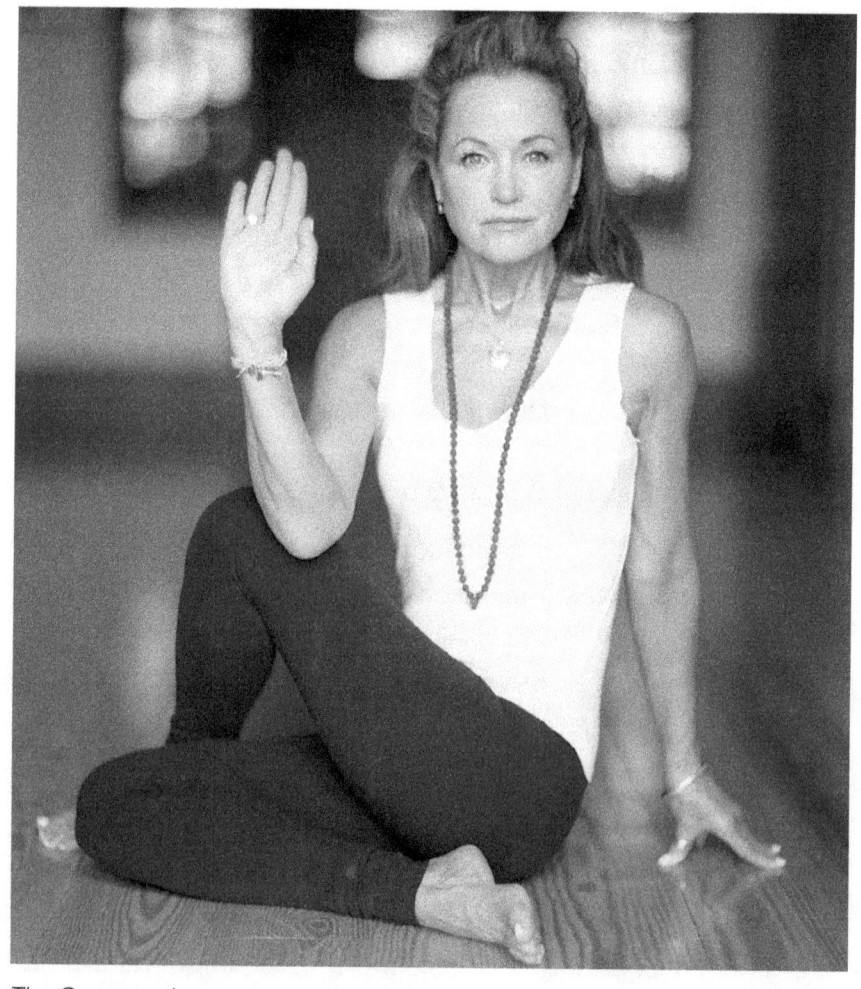

The Command

These all follow the descriptive formats used in the Yoga Practice Appendices for this book and my complete Yoga Manual, which sequentially note the elements that are "Foundational" (basic and used again and again), "Day to Day" (those most applicable, and used, in day-to-day Yoga practice), and "Sessional" (those that are parts of Kriyas, prescribed sessions, and the like).

1. Foundational Knowledge of Body Postures (Asanas) and Hand and Finger Positions (Mudras)

Yoga Postures (Asanas)

Your Yoga practice will include well over one hundred Yoga Postures ("Asanas") used together in innumerable combinations. The most instructional way to organize these, not in any way that is "official" to Yoga, but in a way that will immediately give a sense of both their variety and interrelationship is to simply group them by the general body positions from which they are initiated. In sum, that is:

- Yoga Asanas initiated from the *Standing* Position,
- Yoga Asanas initiated from the various *Sitting* Positions,
- Yoga Asanas initiated from the various *Lying* Positions, and
- Yoga Asanas initiated from "being on *All Fours*" (Hands and Knees).

This is the landscape that you'll become familiar with, across the innumerable names and terms that are now familiar to millions worldwide because of Yoga's popularity—cat-cow, downward dog, plough, fish, cobra, bow, crow, warrior, and so on.

Hand and Finger Poses (Mudras)

Positions of the hands and fingers used both in Yoga postures (Asanas) and with Meditation and Mantra are diverse and of ancient heritage. They are called Mudras. They will be introduced throughout the practices in this book and are detailed more in the special Yoga Practice Appendices assembled for this book—and in my Yoga Manual. To familiarize you immediately with some of the most often used of these, I describe below the most well-known mudra often associated with meditation.

- *Gyan Mudra* [aka "Gesture of Consciousness" or "Seal of Knowledge"]: Gyan Mudra is perhaps the most well-known mudra because it is portrayed widely in art and statuary. The hand is held open, palms up, with the tip of the thumb joining with the tip of the index finger (to form a circle). Gyan Mudra has two variations—active and passive. In "active," the index finger is tucked under the end of the thumb; in "passive," the tips of the thumb and index finger are touching directly. The passive version is the most widely used.

2. Foundational Knowledge of the Breathwork (Pranayama) and Mantra

Breathwork (Pranayama)

Breathwork (Pranayama) in Yoga is often referred to as "the science of breath" because ancient knowledge of breathing in Yogic practice is very precise. Yogic breathing techniques are diverse, ranging from variations of the depth and length of inhalations and exhalations (from "Simple" or "Natural" breathing to "Long Deep Breathing") to more precisely directed techniques ("Breath of Fire," "Alternate Nostril Breathing," and so on). It's important that I acquaint you, right away, with the basic concept surrounding breathing.

- *Inhalation and Exhalation*: Yogic practice recognizes three regions of the body involved in our capacities for breath-related work: the abdominal area ("Abdominal Breath"—from the pelvis to the bottom of the ribs), the chest area ("Chest Breath"—from the bottom of the rib cage to top of the rib cage), and neck and head area ("Clavicular Breath"—from the upper rib to base of the skull). In Yoga practices herein and in my Yoga Manual, I acquaint you in much more detail with various specific breathing techniques.

Mantra

To the breathing techniques of Yoga are added a wonderfully diverse area of activities emerging from our species ability to "sing." All the Yogas are acknowledged as "Naad" Yogas—the Yogas of *sound*. And, in the Yogas, this use of our human ability to "sing" is the world of Mantra. Mantra not only involves the sound itself, and the act of "singing" or "chanting," but it also includes an additional mystical element because of the ancientness of these Mantra words and what they have carried in our collective consciousness and subconsciousness over millennia. It is important to mention this upfront in a foundational way so Mantra can be more specifically elaborated as this book unfolds. You will learn more about it initially when you are introduced to "Tuning In," the way all Kundalini Yoga practices begin. There, right away, you will utilize the ancient *Adi Mantra* (meaning "primal sound"). Later in this book, I provide a complete section on "Yoga and Sound – Meditation, Mantra and Music."

3. Foundational Knowledge of the Bandhas (Locks) and the Chakras

Because the Yoga cosmology of the Chakras is fundamental to Kundalini Yoga, I must also familiarize you right away with the Bandhas (or "Locks"). The Bandhas (or Locks) are uses of the muscles in various areas around the spine to channel the energies of Yogic practice, especially the "Kundalini energy." For Yoga practice purposes, the Bandhas (or Locks) require a detailed description, which I provide herein as Foundational Yoga Practice Appendix 2 and also in my Yoga Manual. To understand the Bandhas (Locks), which are used throughout Kundalini Yoga practice, we must also refer to the Chakras, which were introduced to you in the previous section on Yoga Cosmology. Below, I will summarize the Bandhas (Locks), with their names, pronunciations, and most fundamental relations to the Chakra system. The detailed explanations in my Yoga Manual are also available to you as we go deeper into Yoga practices.

- *Rootlock* (aka *Mulbandh*) [pronounced "mool bond"]: Rootlock (*Mulbandh*) involves the first, second, and third chakras. Its application is described in detail in this book's Appendix 2 and in my Yoga Manual. During Yoga practice, the Teacher advises regularly on the application and use of Rootlock.
- *Diaphragm Lock* (aka *Uddiyana Bandha*) [pronounced "oo-di-yana bonda"]: Diaphragm Lock (*Uddiyana Bandha*) serves the solar plexus and the heart chakra. The diaphragm is utilized both for Yoga postures and in chanting. Diaphragm lock is described in detail in this book's Appendix 2 and in my Yoga Manual and the Teacher also advises regularly regarding its application.
- *Neck Lock or Chin Lock* (aka *Jalandhara Bandha*) [pronounced "jah-lon-DAR-ah bonda"]: Neck Lock (*Jalandhara Bandha*) is the most basic and most generally applied lock. It especially serves the throat chakra and, since located in the strategic region between the torso and head, is important to all the higher chakras. The Teacher advises often regarding Neck Lock, as it involves finessed movements of the neck, chin, head, breastbone, and chest.
- *Great Lock* (aka *Maha Bandha*) [pronounced "MAH-ha bonda"]: Great Lock (*Maha Bandha*) involves the application of all three of the Bandhas ("Locks") nearly simultaneously in a

quick sequence, thus providing the results of all the Bandhas at once. Normally, Rootlock is applied first, and when it is relaxed, the Diaphragm is then applied. When it is relaxed the Neck Lock is then applied and relaxed. The Teacher always advises further on the sequences and durations for these applications, as noted in far more detail in the section on Chakras and Bandhas (Locks) in this book's Appendix 2 and in my Yoga Manual.

For much more detail on both the Bandhas (Locks) and their relationships to specific Chakras, see the entries in my Yoga Manual.

4. Foundational Knowledge of the Elements of Yoga Daily Practice ("Foundational," "Day to Day," and "Sessional")

Of course, the foundation of the Yoga practice that works for you will be up to you, and part of the great adventure. As teachers are fond of saying: "No one initiates you. You initiate yourself." Certainly, there is no daily practice that is going to work for you—truly work, at the deepest level—than the one that you choose. And, it may be a *process* because, as I'll say more later in "Gauging Your Progress...," Yogic practice has an ingenious, if not truly mystical, way in which we are aware of our growth, aware of epiphany after epiphany, and can well gauge our progress.

There are basic components to the practice you will build, and these may vary with the many options within Yoga, across all its varieties. Each of these is rooted in one of the ancient traditions. So, the number and sequence of the components may vary. In Kundalini Yoga, from the great Sikh traditions, which is the one of my background, Yogic life includes nine components I established earlier.

- *Mantras* (that is, "chants")

- *Prayers* (that is, traditional prayer, but especially from the ancient Wisdom Traditions)
- *Mudras* (that is, positions of the hands and fingers)
- *Drishti* (that is, considerations of focus or gaze)
- *Bandhas* (that is, "Locks" of the body's various muscles for specific purposes of guiding energy)
- *Breathwork* (or "Pranayama") (that is, breath-related attention and exercises)
- *Asanas* (that is, various of the traditional "postures" of Yoga)
- *Meditation* (that is, immersion in silence or guided consciousness exercises)
- *Kriyas* (that is, prescribed sequences of all the above)

These aspects are all interconnected, of course: asanas (or postures), positions of the hands and fingers (mudras), meditation, breathwork, and the arrangement of these into sequences (kriyas). With this comes specific attention to details of asanas, breathwork, and kriyas—like focus and gaze (drishti), the bandhas (or locks), and then addition of prayer and mantra.

Each of these will figure into your daily practice. It's likely that they will also diverge to comprise how you practice by yourself, how you practice with a community, or how you practice when you are taking further instruction from a Teacher.

This is why I organize my Yoga Manual and related teaching programs in three stages: Foundational, Day to Day, and Sessional. The Foundational guides are about the elements that you will use over and over, every day, and from which you will build out many more options. The Day to Day guides contain all these latter options which, if they were enumerated completely across the traditions, would number in the hundreds. Then come the kriyas, the sequences of the hundreds of elements in the nine categories above. That is where the Sessional guides come in. The Sessional guides are really guides to kriyas, and, in the Yoga traditions, there are thousands of these. In this book, and my Yoga Manual, Yoga practices have been drawn from these larger Foundational, Day to Day, and Sessional guides as best fits the need of the inspirational message I am conveying and the practice I have attached to it. The descriptive formats in my Yoga Manual and those published by *Light on Light Magazine*, Sacred U. or Humanity's Stream are all similar.

Thus, in Yoga practices herein, I will be including many foundational elements. You can think of them as the roots and trunk of the tree of your growing practice. These will feature most of the basic and fundamental activities and concepts of Kundalini Yoga practice. Then, you will have sequences that are normally a part of day-to-day practice. These are much like the developing branches of your tree where you are building out, through many limbs and branches, the entire landscape of Yogic practice and growing understanding. The ultimate component will be kriyas (each of which are like a "Session" of a Sessional Guide). Instruction and experience with sessions (kriyas) is essential because kriyas are ordered in precise sequences—for an important reason. Every kriya serves a specific function and has a specific goal. Kriyas are then also sequenced into elaborate "sessions." These also have a specific goal regarding health, wellness, well-being, and so on. You can think of these sequences of "kriyas" and sessions as all the varieties of foliage and blossoms you can create with your growing tree of Yogic practice.

Opening Daily Practices: Warming Up and Tuning In

Let me acquaint you now with the traditional "Warming Up and Tuning In" that begins every Yoga practice in the Sikh Kundalini Yoga tradition. This "Warming Up and Tuning In" is detailed completely in Yoga Practice Appendix 3 herein. But, briefly, the sequence is as follows.

Beginning in "Easy Pose" the most common sitting position in Yoga, the hands are drawn together in front of you, palm to palm, and the palms are briskly rubbed back and forth as if to warm them. This livens the arms and body and gets you ready for Yoga practice. Then, the hands are drawn together, palm to palm, in front of the chest at heart level, as in the gesture of "Namaste" or Eastern bowing–which is called "Prayer Pose."

In the Kundalini Yoga tradition, tune-in is done with two short Ancient Chants (mantras) from the Sikh tradition. The language is Gurmukhi, but you'll easily become accustomed to it from the Teacher and more familiar students demonstrating it, and with the English transliterations of the words, as in the Yoga Practice Appendices herein.

The opening Mantra is known in the ancient traditions as the *Adi Mantra* (meaning "primal sound"), sometimes colloquially also called simply *"Ong Namo."* Of course, the Teacher will often demonstrate but the transliteration makes it easy: *Ong Namo, Guru Dev Namo*, pronounced as detailed in the Appendix. It is repeated three times, or as instructed. The literal translation is "I bow to the Creative Wisdom, I bow to the Divine Teacher," meaning, of course, both within and without. This tuning in connects you to both Source and Self.

This mantra is followed by a second short mantra, the "Mantra of the Heart," also repeated three times or as instructed. This mantra is also often called, from its first line: *Aad Guray Nameh*, pronounced as detailed in this book's Appendix 3. It is a prayer for protection and success. Translated through all four of its lines, it means: "I bow to Primal Wisdom; I bow to the Wisdom of the Ages; I bow to True Wisdom; I bow to the great unseen Wisdom."

You can then move into your daily practice, session practice, or whatever the case may be.

Daily Practice: Breathing (Pranayama) Elements

Previously, in "Foundational Knowledge of the Breathwork (Pranayama) and Mantra," I acquainted you with the Yoga cosmology of breathing. In Kundalini, there are some foundational breathing elements, used over and over again, and in combination with other asanas. Let me mention them right away.

The first is called "Breath of Fire" (*Agni Pran*), and it is quite important to Kundalini Yoga. Breath of Fire is a rapidly pulsed breathing, from either the nose or from the mouth, as instructed. It is rather like "panting," which can be employed at many different rates. Often, it is learned first by mimicking a dog panting, with the mouth open and the tongue out, but when familiar, it becomes a more natural, but strong, pulsed breath. It can be learned comfortably by simply having a strong out-breath which makes the in-breath almost automatic. It is important to learn Breath of Fire accurately so that it can serve its Yogic purposes, and the Teacher can help with that.

Other often used day to day Breathing (*Pranayama*) elements include long deep breathing and alternate nostril breathing. These are described in detail in this book's Appendix 3.

With these introductions and preparatory hints, let's now move from inspiration and introduction to basic elements of Yoga Practice combined with Inspired Messages. The efficacy, indeed, the grace, of Yoga is reflected in the fact that for every real-life situation there is a Yoga practice that addresses it directly. So, in the eight entries that follow, I have selected inspiring life messages and combined them with a provenly effective Yoga practice. I think you will find that each message is "special" and that the insights and inspirations within each are then further amplified by the direct addition of a specific Yoga practice.

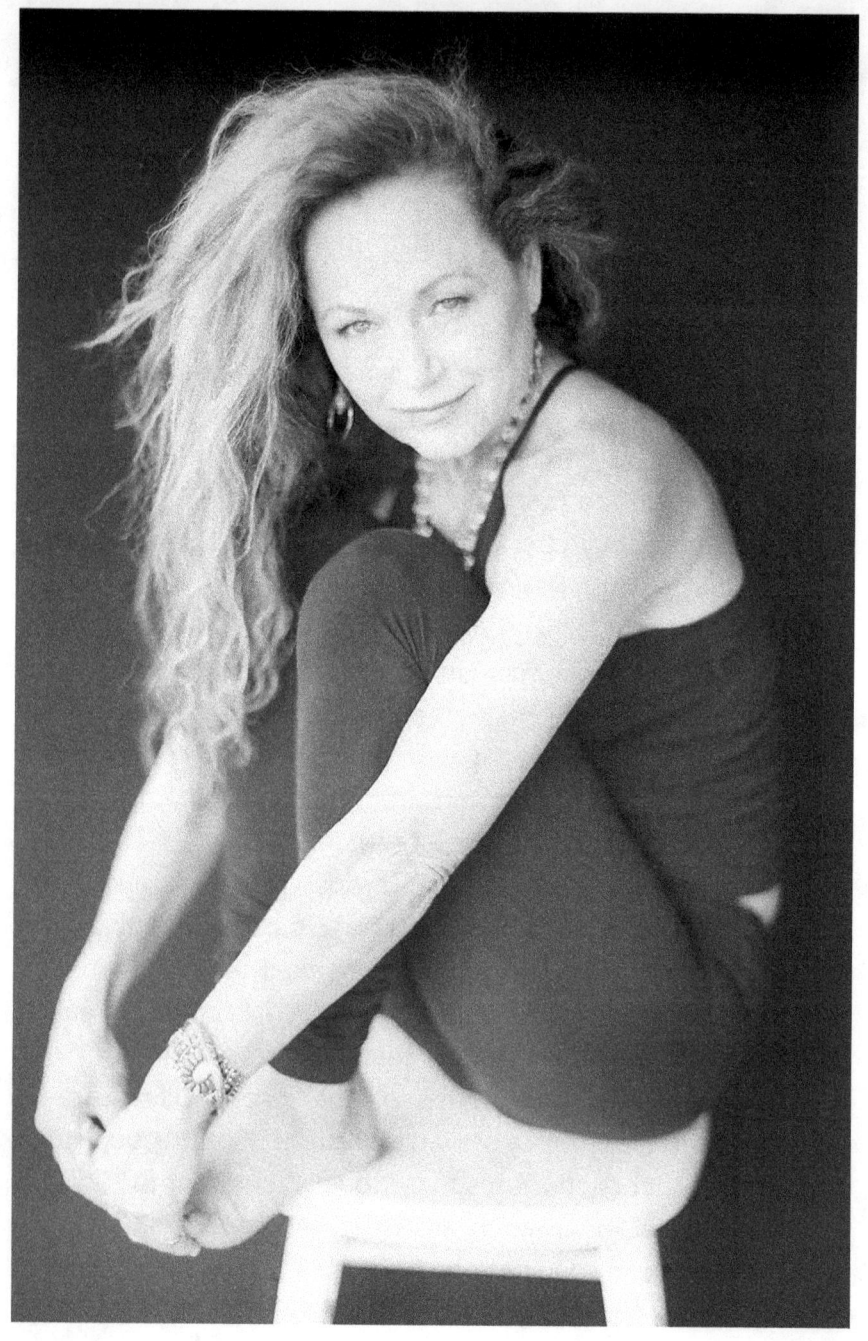

Connection

INSPIRED MESSAGES
with Yoga Practices

Let me introduce you now to the Inspirations and Practices I have specially selected for this book. These Inspired Messages, combined with specific Yoga practices, can now put your entry into Yoga practice and lifestyle into high gear. Below are the inspired topics I'll be addressing and their companion Yoga practices. Each of the Yoga practices is explained in detail in this book's Yoga Practice Appendices as well as in my Yoga Manual.

In enjoying these practices, you'll be experiencing some of the most tried and true Yoga Kriyas—sequences of practice—that the wisdom and skills of Yoga's millennial history have to offer. They are also ones that have been key to my life. Featured are:

- Our Opportunity to Connect with the Divine
  – *with Kriya for Growing Closer to the Divine*
- Healing Grief
  – *with Balancing the Five Tattvas (SaTaNaMa, Kriya for Instinctual Self and Sat Kriya) and Ancient Kriyas for Healing Grief (Pittra Kriya, Shuni Mudra and Superman Pose)*
- Becoming Zero Over and Over Again
  – *with Kriya for Elevation*
- Awakening the Ten Bodies
  – *with Kriya for Awakening the Ten Bodies*
- Interiors and Exteriors
  – *Balancing, with Nabhi Kriya with Prana and Apana*
- How to Stay Natural
  – *with Sat Kriya*

- Gauging Your Progress and Preventing Burnout
  – *with Meditation Against Burnout*
- Grace and Gracefulness in Transitions
  – *with Nahbi Kriya*

In these accounts, you will recognize issues and challenges that came to the fore during the COVID pandemic we all faced together—and all that came with it. You'll recognize challenges that each of us face across day-to-day life. You'll see the role that Yoga inspiration and Yoga practice steps into in facing challenges—nurturing us and giving us that promised "Way Out" of whatever the "rabbit hole" might be.

Beyond the individual level, you'll witness the healing, energizing—and ultimately Awakening—role that Yoga plays all across the world in providing a "way" for millions. In critical areas of our global culture, Yoga communities do crucial service work in the realms of health and wellness, especially for the critical needs of women and children, water and sanitation, agriculture, workplace equality and safety, and diverse arenas of social justice. This work goes on around the world, and very often on a voluntary, community basis.

These acts of care, concern, and kindness all reflect the implications of the superlative ethics and values of Yogic teachings themselves. On a global level, we see the importance of the well-being that is available through Yogic practice and how potent it is in the process of personal and global awakening. So, as you enjoy these inspirations and associated practices, I hope you can also appreciate what a grand and cosmic transformative process of which you are a part. Use that inspiration to the fullest in your own pursuit of the fruits of Yoga and the Yogic life.

Intention

As we begin this journey of inspiration and practice, let's become aware of our Intentions. Going directly to this point often solves so many things and speeds up the process of progress and transformation. This is why I often ask people, "What is your intention?" It's like asking where on a target they want to shoot an arrow. Be clear. That's what's important. When you are clearly aware of your intentions, you'll start to notice how this perks up the clarity in everything you do—when to slow down, when to take that break, or even when to nap to refresh yourself so you can be at your best for yourself and others. When you do this, you'll start to sense when you're "off" and when you're "on," when you're balanced and when you're not. If you take care of *yourself*, you can really be available in a loving and kind way to others.

It's a natural reciprocity—one that is built into all of nature, and our inner Nature too—that we want to share with others, and them with us. It's so natural that it's the origin of The Golden Rule: "Do unto others as you would have them do unto you," or "Elicit the best in others and, thereby, in yourself."

When you think about it, all this is really an exercise in listening, and I/we will talk about listening in many other places in this book. "Communication" is back and forth, so it's both giving and receiving.

When you start living this way, you'll notice that your "intuition" develops more and more, because intuition is a refined form of listening. The Yogic practice and lifestyle are all about this kind of deep listening. It's actual participation in the subtle realms of our shared reality and what the universe is made of. Everything we do in Kundalini Yoga—all the refined relationships between the Chakras and the energy bodies, and on and on, are a part of this network of fine-grained interrelations.

From the largest perspective, one could say Yoga and the entire Yogic experience are like a Friend you can listen to. You'll find that your practice provides messages about your progress, what you need, what's up, and what's next.

I can say that I have made my Yoga my best friend, and now she speaks louder than I do! And she's also a really good tour guide, about which we'll say much more. So, let's begin.

OUR OPPORTUNITY TO CONNECT WITH THE DIVINE

– with Kriya for Growing Closer to the Divine
[Yoga Practice Appendix 4]

We may not think of it, let alone realize it, but in our life on this planet, we have this unique opportunity to connect with the Divine. Think about it for a moment. It's *huge*, isn't it? From all the problems we appear to have, and all the twists and turns in our lives, we have, in any moment, the opportunity to connect with the Divine.

Even if we didn't believe in the Divine, or thought that we didn't believe in the Divine, the mention of this possibility to connect with it is a life-changing realization.

This actually explains "devotion." What else is devotion except someone taking advantage of their opportunity to connect with the Divine? If this is true, you'd think you'd have to be crazy not to seize this opportunity (*Carpe diem!* [Seize the day!]).

After all, thinking of it another way, what else is unhappiness than feeling separate, feeling alone, feeling there is no meaning to anything?

Practitioners of this kind of deep Devotion say that the connection to the Divine happens automatically when the right tools are used. Do it, and it happens. We can understand this by thinking of flowers. If someone puts a beautiful rose in front of you, the message that it is beautiful comes automatically. It doesn't take analysis to decide whether the rose is beautiful or not; it just is. And it's right there, in front of you.

So, the tool kit of Kundalini Yoga is full of these kinds of flowers, with the one that is the most obvious being the music.

The music of Yogic lifestyle, chant, and devotional music, tells you automatically, simply by what it does to you, that it is a bridge to this other state—the state of the Divine—which is about spirit, positivity, gratitude, beauty, peace, and well-being.

And if it brings these things to you, those traits of spirit, positivity, gratitude, beauty, peace, and well-being are replacing the clutter that's accumulated in your body and soul. So, it's a cleansing that goes on, and, because you identify with the message of the music and say that big "Yes" to it, those qualities are replacing the lower, gross, and mundane accumulations of life so you can not only feel cleansed and comforted but also, yes, connected with the Divine.

This connection is so automatic to who we are that it explains what Yogis say, that mantra always serves the need of the time—it fits the need of our life, right now. And if this is true, it explains why it becomes a lifestyle. Who doesn't want to feel this connection as often as possible? It is a part of our birthright, which is why we both seek it, and find it.

- Enjoy the Related Practice: *Kriya for Growing Closer to the Divine* [Yoga Practice Appendix 4 where I give an additional introduction to this Kriya]

HEALING GRIEF
– with Balancing the Five Tattvas (SaTaNaMa, Kriya for Instinctual Self and Sat Kriya) and Ancient Kriyas for Healing Grief (Pittra Kriya, Shuni Mudra and Superman Pose)
[Yoga Practice Appendix 5]

The need for healing—indeed rebirth—after human tragedy is as old as the human story itself. Such is the recognition of human suffering that it is part of both the Four Noble Truths and the Three Marks of Existence of our great Eastern traditions. It is also central to the incarnational theologies—suffering and resurrection—of the West. We need only to see the cycle of Easter each year for that message to be driven home.

In the Four Noble Truths, the first "Dukkha" (or "truth of life") is recognized as the perpetuity of such conditions as pain, suffering, unhappiness, and dissatisfaction. In the Three Marks of Existence, these conditions join impermanence and non-self (our inherent insecurity about identity) as the third great truth. It is from all of these that we naturally seek rebirth. This process requires in us a deep sense of our innate self-worth and our birthright to a better, healthier life. Familiar with this inevitable process, Jesus himself said: "unless a grain of wheat fall into the ground and die, it abideth alone; but if it die, it bringeth forth much fruit" (John 12: 24). In all the traditions, it is the rebirth to a new life, a new health, that is the goal and fruit of transformation.

The 2020-2021 global COVID pandemic appears iconic, even archetypal, in its summoning of this pattern from calamity to rebirth. We remember a similar pandemic of the 14th Century which, while tragically killing nearly one-third of the population of Europe and Asia at the time, also ushered in The Renaissance. The rebirth of The Renaissance then led to unparalleled new invention, advancement, and prosperity for humankind. Similarly, the 2020-2021 global pandemic brought the reality of uncertainty, fear, illness, suffering, and death square into the faces of millions worldwide. We may not—indeed, perhaps we cannot—fully comprehend the cosmic "reasons" for such calamity, but we do know that to complete the epic cycle, we must now reconcile, rejuvenate, and heal. Kundalini Yoga—the Yoga of awareness—provides ancient technologies for this destined healing, this delicate process of moving from grief and loss back to the certain path of our rebirth and Awakening.

During the COVID pandemic, particularly through my opportunities to work with the United Nations International Day of Yoga, and then to carry those programs forward online through Sacred Stories, Humanity's Stream, and others, I was able to bring these healing Yoga techniques to thousands. I will tell you more about these activities when I come to the topic of Rebirth, but first, I want to share these essential teachings about healing grief.

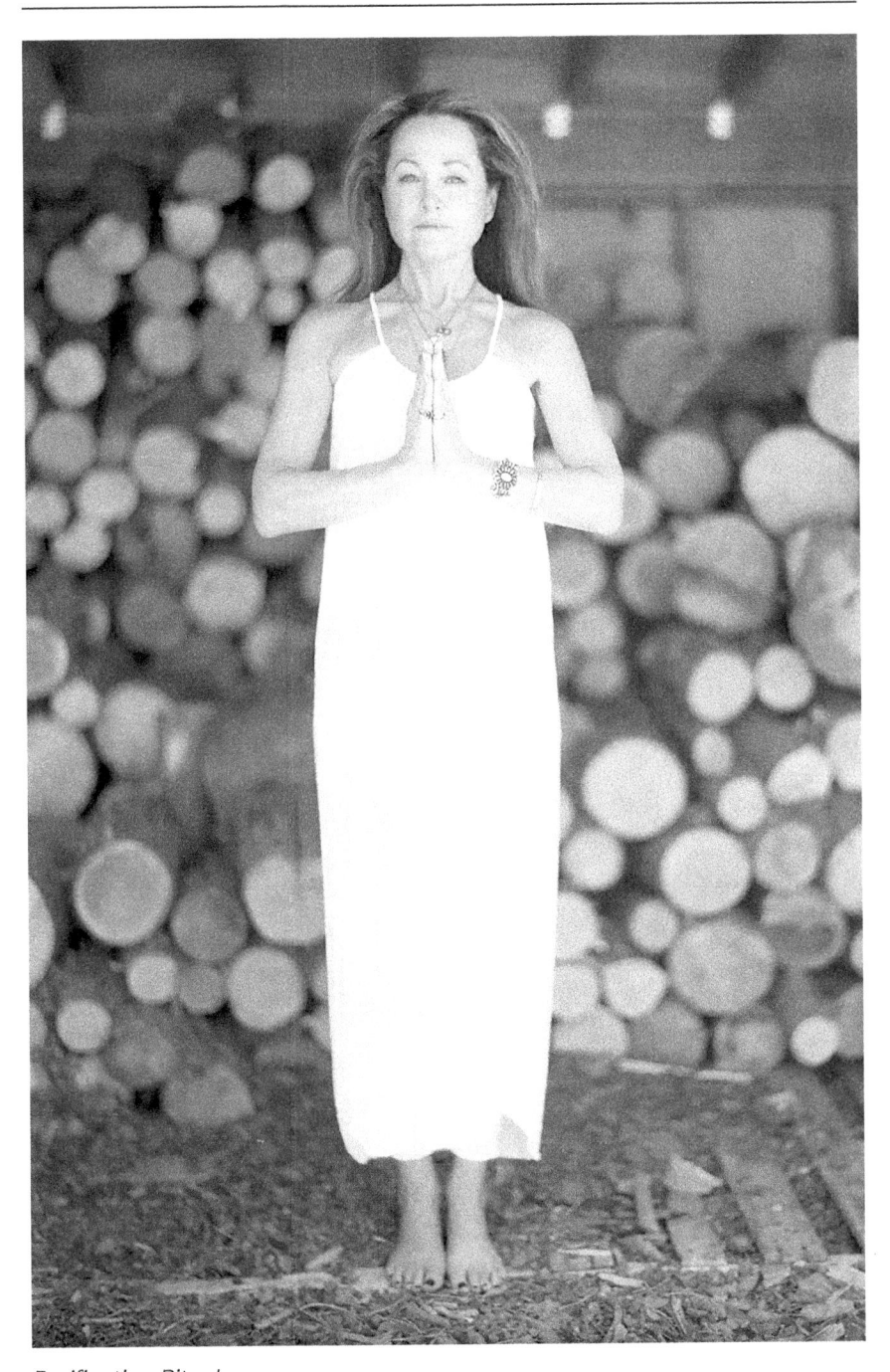

Purification Rituals

Kundalini Yoga and Healing Grief

Grief is only the first layer of trauma. We store grief under our anger, resentment, destruction, and the way we speak to ourselves. It is so important to understand the layers of grief so we can release them.

These ancient programs, which have proven themselves over and over, include those for the Healing Grief process outlined in detail in the Spiritual Practices Appendices herein.

The first part is "Getting the Body Out of Distress." The second is "Balancing the Five Tattvas" (the five states of matter and spirit), which utilizes the ancient kriyas "SaTaNaMa," "Kriya for Instinctual Self," and "Sat Kriya." The third part concludes with the "Ancient Kriyas for Healing Grief," comprised of "Pittra Kriya," the "Shuni Mudra," and what has become known as the "Superman Pose." Here is how those work:

Getting the Body Out of Distress

To address the body's distress, we need to understand that grief, anxiety, worry, fear, concern, etc. are not just experiences in our psyches and emotions. Because we are holistic organisms of spirit and body, all psychic and emotional elements are also deeply embedded in our bodies. In Yoga, such stress is seen as a "frozen" state. It needs to be released with relaxation of both body and spirit. Because we are holistic organisms, addressing grief first requires that we make the body comfortable. The body needs to know, by conscious thought and also from our deepest subtle energies, that it is loved. Not only is this important to the initial recognition and calming of the body, but it also creates the environment for a whole-systems approach to the role of healing grief, trauma, and regret necessary for us being free to begin the transformative processes that we are undertaking.

Balancing the Five Tattvas

With the body calmed and knowing that it is loved, we can continue to address balancing across all the senses. In the ancient tradition, and using the Sanskrit terms from Yoga cosmology, this is the process for "Balancing the Five Tattvas." Ancient wisdom discovered five qualities of our senses in the world and our senses of the world. After quieting and relaxing the body, we want to balance these five essential ways that we all sense in, and of, the world.

The ancient traditions called these five elements or tattvas "Earth, Water, Fire, Air, and Ether." Today, we know ether as Consciousness. Further, we recognize the intertwining of earth, air, fire, and water as the essential "states of matter"—gasses, liquids, and solids—and their combustions ("fire") that form both our bodies and the entire universe. That's quite a lesson, as I've said, in how holistic our bodies really are. They are truly stardust—as the astronomers regularly remind us.

The kriyas I'm describing here are ones time-tested and proven through millennia for addressing trauma, loss, and grief by nurturing this balance of the primordial elements of which we are all made.

The Ancient Kriyas for Healing Grief

The final pieces in the toolkit for healing trauma, loss, and grief have long histories across the Wisdom Traditions of the East. The first is "Pittra Kriya." It has an ancient history in the East for healing from calamity, grief, or disaster. The word itself means "ancestor" or "history" and, thus, directly refers to something lost. Ancient Kriyas for grief like these were often practiced in nature, especially by a river, to give the sense of healing with the flowing of time. In Yoga, stress is seen as a "frozen" state. It needs to be released with relaxation of both body and spirit, which is the function of these Kriyas.

Of course, suffering, loss, and tragedy are an inevitable part of the impermanence that marks our lives (the First Noble Truth and Third Mark of Existence) and part of the panorama of change in this process. Inevitably, we move on from grief and tragic loss to return to the path of our birthright, the path to ultimate Awakened life. That path always remains there, even during the darkest times. Because such apparent deaths, but real rebirths, may occur often in our lives, it's important that we understand them and learn from them.

There are a number of lessons here, and they are worth noting. One lesson we learn is that, yes, this dark time *was* a real and calamitous intrusion onto the path of our birthright. But also, we may realize in hindsight that, on this path, there are also sometimes hidden gifts in these tragedies. I've already told you one of those stories in "Failing Better and Succeeding Better," and I will tell you another in "Grace and Gratefulness in Transitions." So, sometimes, we experience these hidden gifts or what is also often called "fierce grace."

Grief and Wisdom

There is more wisdom I want to share about grief, trauma, and loss. It requires that we take a rather cosmic, big picture, look at suffering—and a cosmic look in light of all the wisdom of the ancient teachings of "Truth." Let's first take a look at the meaning of the word "Truth" itself. That definition might seem like a tall order, but the answer is actually a simple one, really just a matter of common sense. We can define truth as simply "something that does not change." It is always the same. Even if we think of the dynamic of change itself, the definition remains true. An example is the "truth" of a waterfall—always changing in dynamic movement, but always the same—verified in a hundred different photos of Niagara Falls that are all still identified as "Niagara Falls." What it is, as dynamic movement, does not change.

So, what is the truth about suffering? A wise teacher recognizes that so much suffering comes from emotions and commotions. So much of our suffering comes from stories—such as "who did what to whom"—and we go round and round about it with our emotions. If we're honest, probably 95% of all of our sufferings are from stories of "who did what to whom" and "he said / she said." They come simply from the emotions and commotions stirred up by stories that we tell.

But what about the other 5%? Well, that 5% of suffering is truly real, but we need to understand why. That 5% is grief and loss—loss or fear of impending loss of a person or place that is loved. That suffering is real because with real love—which is something we innocently give ourselves completely to with real vulnerability—we actually have an "energy loop" or "connection" to the person or place we love. So, when they are taken away from us, there is truly a rupture in the energy field, or loop, that we have with that person or place. The rupture in the shared energy field is real and causes suffering that must have its own rather uncharted course as to resolution and healing. The reality of this relationship of shared energy, with grief and loss, makes our practices for healing grief and loss even more important. So, save your suffering for the big ones.

- Enjoy the Related Practice: *Balancing the Five Tattvas (SaTaNaMa, Kriya for Instinctual Self and Sat Kriya)* and *Ancient Kriyas for Healing Grief (Pittra Kriya, Shuni Mudra and Superman Pose)* [Yoga Practice Appendix 5 where I give an additional introduction to these Practices]

BECOMING ZERO OVER AND OVER AGAIN
– with Kriya for Elevation
[Yoga Practice Appendix 6]

After Healing Grief, the next Inspiration we want to share is the process of elevation and rebirthing—our continual returning to zero over and over again, followed by rebirthing to our destiny of Awakened life.

We've all heard the phrase from a famous poet, "the greatest schemes of mice and men often go awry," or "life is something that happens when you're busy making other plans."

It's natural—and innocent—that people invest in dreams and plans. But the craziest things can go wrong. Sometimes, it's dramatic, like with Christopher Reeve ("Superman") being thrown from a horse and finding himself paralyzed. Other times, it's the loss of a job, a career, or a loved one when "you didn't see it coming."

These are natural occurrences, often with no one to blame. But the truth is they affect the recipient of this "turn-about" profoundly. This is particularly true when the turn-about is a reversal of their entire life plans, or life dreams.

We can learn a lot about the many minor reversals that are likely to happen in our lives from speaking to people who have experienced *big* reversals. Nearly all of them will tell you that, at first (perhaps even for months or years), they felt angry and confused, perhaps even not wanting to live. But, amazingly, they usually all report that, at some point, they realized that since they could not change their situation, there were many possibilities to look at it as an opportunity—an opportunity for something wholly new. They describe it as "a turning point," and some also note that, in order for them to enter into this new opportunity, they had to learn to give themselves a "new permission."

For many, the Yogic pursuit is like this. On multiple levels, people in Yogic practice describe it as a turning point, and often a turning point that led them, as they say, to truly understand themselves and their sense of a "destiny." We might think of this word "destiny" as implying some kind of a "really big deal"—fame, fortune, whatever—but wouldn't happiness itself be enough? Remember, "Happiness is your birthright." That's a really good destiny to start with!

This phenomenon of becoming zero again isn't just about the big results of your life—whether or not your achievement meets the vision of your ultimate goal. Many of us know it's also about perseverance along the way. What's it like when you have a clear feeling about a calling or goal, and even those closest to you are seeing it from their perspective?

If you are truly dedicated to your vision, this brings you to another zero point—no one is supportive, but inside, your Self is telling you that you still have to do your work! You doing things that are new, or in a different way, or in ways that "don't fit in," can bring more than just lack of support. It can sometimes also bring bullying and active resistance against you.

So, when we are in this predicament it's important to go deep and to find the kind of inner compass that gives a sense of not only "our work" but our ability to complete it—to do what you're called to do.

This is "Sadhana"—which is such a gift to this "going deep." Sadhana is the name for the gathering of the Yoga community for meditation and practice, in the very early morning, actually before dawn. Lasting some two and one-half hours, the practitioner, in their own private space, or spaced at intervals among the community, and also being guided by the Teacher, devotes this significant time to "what will land" in this mystical container.

I'm going to be saying much more about Sadhana throughout this book. I will devote an entire chapter ("Sadhana") to its general concept and how it is practiced. Sadhana has so many aspects to it and is such a crucial opportunity for every Yoga practitioner. To begin briefly, let's take a look at the multiple meanings of Sadhana. Sadhana has meanings in more than a half dozen languages among the Great Wisdom Traditions. In its simplest meaning, it is often used as a synonym of "meditation." As a verb, it is used to mean "to form," "to accustom," "to train," or even "to subdue" [the Hinkhoj Hindi-English Dictionary]. In its spiritual usages, it literally means "a means of accomplishing something" and is attributed to "any spiritual exercise that is aimed at progressing towards the very ultimate expression of one's life in this reality" [Wikipedia]. Similar definitions of it—in the spiritual context—include anything that is a tool for your well-being, whereby bondage becomes liberation [Wikipedia] and then elevates to perfection [Collins Dictionary]. And there are many more.

Sadhana really creates an environment in which you can return to the zero point. It creates a nest, or landing zone, into which can drop the inspirations, discernments, and determinations that can allow you to move forward step by step. And, when you have found that support within yourself, it's likely you also will find it from others, that others "will show up" who understand and support your work and vision. But for purposes of this Message, let's concentrate on "that which elevates to perfection" and, thus, the practice that is recommended below.

- Enjoy the Related Practice: *Kriya for Elevation* [Yoga Practice Appendix 6 where I give an additional introduction to this Kriya]

AWAKENING THE TEN BODIES
– with Kriya for Awakening the Ten Bodies
[Yoga Practice Appendix 7]

Sharing with you about Awakening the Ten Bodies provides a wonderful opportunity to speak about my truly fulfilling work with the United Nations International Day of Yoga. With the global pandemic in 2020-21, this work—and Kundalini Yoga's practices for Awakening—became exceedingly important. And, it is work that must continue as our world recovers from one of its most profound historical traumas.

It was Awakening the Ten Bodies that I offered throughout the pandemic, following directly on the Healing Grief practices that I have just shared with you above. A major sharing of these practices was broadcast with the Committee for the International Day of Yoga at the United Nations for the June 21 Yoga Day program for 2020. Because of COVID it was an on-line program—and ultimately reached over 30,000 persons.

I was then able to follow up these important messages and practices from the International Day of Yoga through an online program at SacredStories.com's "Sacred U" and at Humanity's Stream where both programs are now permanently available.

Rebirthing and The International Day of Yoga (or IDY)

Each year, the magazine I host and co-edit—*Light on Light Magazine*—co-creates an annual Yoga Day issue. It is curated by the Committee for the International Day of Yoga at the United Nations (the "UNIDY") and lets people all around the world know what Yoga communities are doing on a global level. 2020 and 2021 were special because of the sudden and unexpected trauma of COVID, the challenges of lockdowns, and then the long healing and recovery period for so many people around the world. The period also was filled with political and social unrest and turmoil—of which we are all aware. Thus, the world's Yoga communities not only had Yoga Day to observe and to celebrate but also to address herculean challenges and traumas. With myriad illnesses, and millions of deaths worldwide, attention to grief and reawakening became paramount.

It was wonderful co-creating these programs with the UN Yoga Day Committee, and I think you will find them inspiring. The program *Light on Light* co-created with the UNIDY combined my practices for Healing Grief with The Awakening of the Ten Bodies. The Yoga Day broadcast program was entitled "Yoga Wisdom for Healing and Peace." Attesting to its compelling relevance in the midst of the global pandemic, the program had over 8,000 online participants when it aired and another 22,000 thereafter. The program was companioned by a presentation from my inspiring yoga colleagues at the Yoga Day committee entitled: "Building a Culture of Diversity." The two programs combined the messages of Yoga and global community. The program began with these words:

> "All beings are born free and equal in dignity and rights. We are endowed with reason and conscience and should act towards one another in a spirit of brotherhood and sisterhood.
>
> While these words are enshrined in the text of the Universal Declaration of Human Rights, they are cornerstones of Yogic philosophy to live by each day. When we respect life, ourselves, each other and our natural world, we open our hearts to our shared humanity and the expansion of connection, unity,

respect, solidarity, compassion and peace. This can lead to ending our own behaviors as well as dismantling institutions that perpetuate intolerance, inequality, discrimination and violence.

Emphasizing spiritual values in this way uplifts the UN's crucial work and the actions of all those dedicated to creating a better world for humanity and our Earth. Recent events have made it clear that no country, no culture can exist on its own, and it is through our unified efforts, by joining together, that we are able to meet pressing needs and provide assistance that affects people in their daily lives.

With the pandemic, the core UNITY message of Yoga and its unparalleled resources for healing and well-being are more important than ever.

Spiritual uplifting that nurtures both body and soul is key, and the Wisdom Schools of Yoga provide major and truly effective rest, respite, rebuilding and rebirth."

This was a perfect introduction to my program of spiritual practice which followed later in the day. I also spoke of rebirth. I remember so well looking into the video cameras and saying, from the depth of my heart:

"There is something we learn about in these times of crisis which is the thing we really should be reaching for all the time. It is a deeper message in our essential Nature. We need to reach for how that Nature, within us, can be acting all the time—not just when a crisis occurs.

In every crisis, there is a rebirthing. In every crisis, there is an opportunity. But it often requires—in us—a new permission, a new permission inside ourselves, a new permission that assures us: "you're healthy;" "you can do this;" "you can trust this;" "this is not something you would have designed for yourself, but it was apparently designed for you."

So, there is a hidden grace in every rebuilding process. From the lessons we learn from each rebuilding, each rebirthing, we come to learn that our life experience on this planet is really about rebuilding everything."

So, with this rich background—which really happened(!)—let's take a look at Awakening the Ten Bodies.

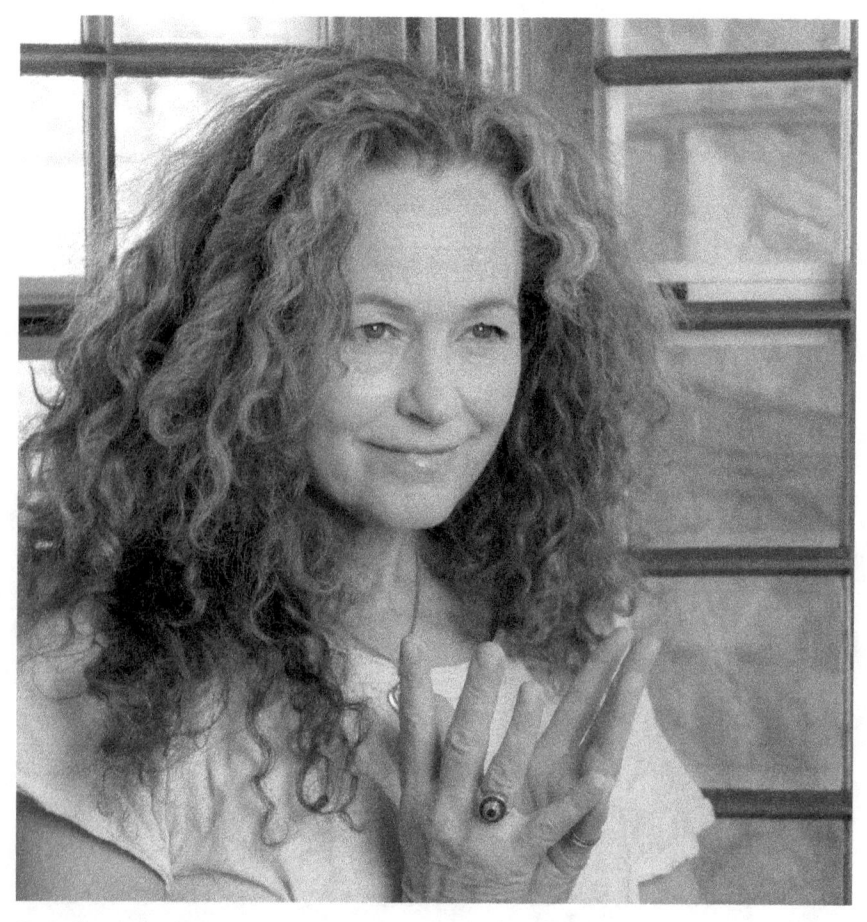

Pure Consciousness

The Ten Bodies

Yogic cosmology teaches that we actually have ten bodies—not just one. They are called the Ten Bodies or the Ten Etheric Bodies since they are actually "Fields" that, together, form the wholeness of our being. Functionally, you could think of the Ten Bodies as the variety of "hats" that "You" actually wear across all the elements of your being, existence, and experience. You might visualize the ten "Fields" simultaneously surrounding the whole of you. As "fields," they don't need to have precise boundaries or shapes. They are dynamic–and always engaged in their own ongoing sustenance *and* further growth. In a way, sensing the Ten Bodies is a bit like listening to music. When you are in your room listening to music, you are clearly aware the music is there, and its content is also clear. However, you wouldn't exactly be able to say "where" the music is in your room or where the various attributes of the music are, e.g., the scherzos or the adagios. Given this dynamism, Yoga cosmology speaks about each of the bodies by noting their various attributes, elements, senses, or characteristics, which help you to understand, and sense, their reality.

The First Body Is the "Soul Body"

As you might imagine, it implies the core of your being, *your* unique part of the wider infinite—in that sense, the deepest root of your identity. As such, it is also the core of your creativity, where your being and your doing synergize. As you have likely also guessed, it is thus aligned with the reality of your Heart. It is *already* in effortless flow with the Divine and, thus, is also the seat of your birthright to Awakened life. When blocked, your Soul Body may cause you to feel separate, uncertain, or tentative, seeking ideas and stories to hang onto rather than acting from the surety of your deepest nature. Balancing of the Soul Body is addressed by the practices of Awakening the Ten Bodies.

The Second Body Is Our Negative, or Protective, Mind

This body is naturally attuned to our animate life. It is the one that senses dangers, advises caution, and examines the "downsides" of decisions we might make or directions we might take. This body actually cares for us by providing this protective capacity. While this caring is admirable and necessary, when imbalanced, this same protective mode may cause us to live too narrowly and prevent us from the courageous embracing and reaching out for our very birthright—our belonging with, and being of, the Divine. So, some growth and mastery is needed to entune this second body with that of the other minds—the positive and neutral. We need that full balance to best serve our ultimate destiny and birthright. These balancing needs are addressed through the practices of Awakening the Ten Bodies.

The Third Body Is Our Positive, or Expansive, Mind

In a way, this body is the seat of your "can do" energy. Its nature is to brim with optimism, vision–thinking big, and reaching out courageously with creativity and will to succeed at making the best of every possible situation. At its best, Positive Mind is truly the driver to help you move toward your destiny in Awakening. This third body is also the seat for fulfillment and fun. But balance here is important. This is because the Third Body is the flipside of the Negative (or Protective) Mind. The two need to work in tandem for what's "just right" for you. You don't want to flip back and forth between optimism and fear, yes and no. You don't want to be careless or act foolishly from over-optimism. As I said earlier, when I acquainted you with Davy Crockett's famous motto, you want to be sure you're on track first, and *then* go ahead. The practices of Awakening the Ten Bodies help you to attain this balance and all the advantages of your Positive Mind.

The Fourth Body Is the Neutral, or Meditative, Mind

This Fourth Body is like having a compass for balancing the pros and cons of both the Positive and Negative minds! That certainly testifies to the design genius of Source. Also known as Meditative Mind, Neutral Mind is our state that—from a calm, neutral base—sees the big picture around us and helps to accurately gauge and discern. Acting from that sense of surety and calm, it increases our productivity because we are not distracted by emotion and commotion. Neutral Mind is truly a seat of our natural intuition and innate wisdom. From this center of calm, one can readily act with love and compassion, seeing truly from the Heart. Without Neutral Mind, or when it is out of balance, we can be bouncing back and forth between the positive and the negative and not sure of ourselves. With it, we have our inherent sense of balance. The practices of Awakening the Ten Bodies help us to experience this Neutral Meditative Mind which is so key to a fully Awakened life.

The Fifth Body Is Our Physical Body

Conventionally, we've often thought this was the only body we have! It is our physical, material form. But as we also have learned already from Yoga cosmology, it is perfectly designed for our destiny, which is our birthright for Awakened life. In our lives on this planet at this time, it is actually the material temple that houses our soul. The physical body also teaches us about the unity and entwined organization of life. It is an ecosystem in itself made up of thousands of elements all cooperating together. Understanding this, we realize that the body is a vehicle for our birthright in Awakened consciousness. The body is—in that sense—also a servant on our path to Awakened life. If not understood, or if imbalanced, the physical body may be forgotten in its divine role, and mistreated and abused, leading to all kinds of physical illnesses and maladies.

The Sixth Body Is the Arcline

The arcline is a very personalized energy field, much like the conventional idea of a "halo," and functions in our most intimate perceptions and communications. The fields of the arcline are intricately linked with the Sixth Chakra (the Third Eye Chakra) and our glandular and nervous systems and are central to our spiritual perceptions and knowing. The arcline differs between the sexes. Both men and women have an arcline, or halo-like energy field, that runs across the brow and hairline from ear to ear. But women have a second arcline that extends across their chests, from nipple to nipple. You can imagine the intimacy of this arcline in the connection of mother and child. The arcline is essential to our perceptions and our deepest levels of knowing. In alignment with the energies of the arcline, the practices of Awakening the Ten Bodies heighten the activities of the pituitary gland, nervous system, and Sixth Chakra (or Third Eye), all central in Awakened life.

The Seventh Body Is the Auric Body

The Auric Body, well known to many as the "Aura," is an electromagnetic Field—some three to ten feet in expanse—around the body. It is readily detected by modern scientific instruments. Spiritually, it is recognized as being connected to a sense of healthy life force and strength of well-being, and, in science, to a healthy immune system. In Yoga cosmology, it is associated with the "Eighth Chakra"—Soul Star or Star Chakra—that occurs above the body's Seventh Chakra—"Crown Chakra"—and, thus, those highest centers of consciousness and Awakening. The practices of Awakening the Ten Bodies provide potent support for the development, nurturing, and elevation of the Auric Body.

The Eighth Body Is the Pranic Body

This body is deeply connected to the dynamics of our breathing and what breathing means both physically and spiritually. As such, it is also key to our degrees of physical and spiritual health and the strength of our presence and well-being. It is intimately involved in the interactions of etheric energy on our inbreaths and outbreaths and, in that, also reflects the internal balances of our masculine and feminine natures. Connecting directly to our degrees of physical health, energy, and, thus, even self-esteem, all Pranayam practices, and especially those of Awakening the Ten Bodies, aid in the sustenance and elevation of the Pranic Body.

The Ninth Body Is the Subtle Body

You might imagine that the Subtle Body is much like the core software in our body/spirit where all of our "files" are contained—not only the deepest senses of self, but also our "antennas and radar" for connection to all the subtle energies of the cosmos. As such, it is also the field that, in Yoga cosmology, connects to our "Akashic Record," which itself connects to the wider Akashic Records of the cosmos. You will find, in even the most conservative definitions of "Akashic Record," something like this:

> A record of all the events, actions, and thoughts that have ever occurred or ever will (both individually and cosmically), all carried, and contained, by the "Akasha." The Akasha is a field of encoded vibrations that carry specific imperishable information much like a radio or television wavefield from which your receiver can retrieve and display specific information.

Reference to the Akashic Record occurs across nearly all Eastern traditions, many Western mystical traditions, and also in the Theosophy and Anthroposophy of more recent times. Quite beyond these rather grand aspects of the Subtle Body, in day-to-day life, it is key to our senses of things, our feelings of well-being, and our abilities to deeply enjoy such things as the arts and the beauty of nature.

The Tenth Body Is the Radiant Body

You might imagine that the Tenth Body, the Radiant Body, is the seat of your birthright for Awakened Life and how you would shine from that summit. It is the deepest seat of your natural self-worth and natural divinity and also the seat of the energy that drives you toward, and forward with, your True Nature. If you've ever been around someone who captivated you with an obvious vibration of goodness, love, and nurturing, you were probably reacting to the strength of their radiant body. It is the part of us that, on the spiritual path and journey to our birthright, declares, "There is no fifty-fifty." The practices of Awakening the Ten Bodies nurture, develop, and elevate the Radiant Body.

The Eleventh Body Is Whole Embodiment

The Eleventh Body—or Whole Embodiment—primordially contains all the other Bodies. As such, wrapping them all in one whole, it is like the Primal Sound (the primal "*Naad*" that is the identity of the entire cosmos). As such, it is also the primal or divine "Name"—the Sat Nam—"God and Me, Me and God, are One." It is really your recognition as completion. In the words from the scriptures of the Sikh tradition, the well-spring of Kundalini Yoga—from the words of the *Siri Guru Granth Sahib*:

> "When the God in you, and the human in you are in parallel unisonness, then you are an 11. You have no duality, you have divine vision, and the truth flows from you. You don't have to find anything outside of you. The jewels are all in you—you are rich inside; you have satisfaction and contentment."

With this preparation, you should be able to truly invest and immerse yourself in the practice of Awakening the Ten Bodies. It is not only provided in the Yoga Practice Appendices in this book but also in my Yoga Manual and free in online format at Sacred U. and Humanity's Stream at these links:

- https://courses.sacredstories.com/courses/tenbodies
- https://stream.humanitysteam.org/awakening-the-ten-bodies-with-karuna

Global Rebirthing

Now to put a capstone on the International Day of Yoga which, in 2020 and 2021, the practices of Healing Grief and Awakening the Ten Bodies were such an important part. Globally, Yoga in the modern era has come a long way. Almost everyone is familiar with Yoga today. With this prodigious presence in global popular culture, and deep roots in the heritages of some of the world's greatest Wisdom Traditions, its "tried and true" methods for bringing well-being to body and mind are now employed all around the world. This is quite a change from when, in earlier centuries, Yoga was well known in only a few of our world's cultures.

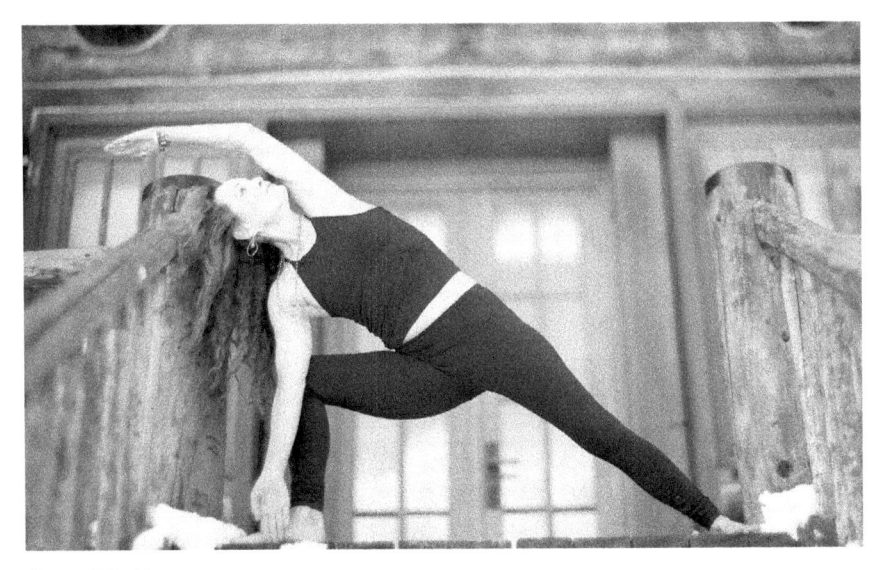

Open My Heart

As recognition of the benefits of Yoga's physical health and meditative components has swept the world, it is no surprise that, in 2014, the United Nations General Assembly proclaimed "The International Day of Yoga," which has been celebrated annually on June 21st ever since. The declaration of The International Day of Yoga provided a unique opportunity to also expand global recognition of the activities of Yoga communities around the world that, every day, serve the critical health and well-being needs of millions of men and women, and especially of children, elders, and the disenfranchised and marginalized.

A global benefit of declaring an International Day of Yoga through the United Nations community has been to facilitate the birth of what has become the International Day of Yoga Committee at the UN. Denise Scotto, Chair of that Committee, has so graced my book with the introduction presented in her Foreword.

The Committee, comprised of members from multiple service organizations from around the world, plays the dual role of not only publicizing the benefits of Yoga itself but also coordinating, and making the rest of the world aware of, the multiple human services that Yoga communities provide all around the world. These include services in clean water, sanitation, health care, safe and prosperous agriculture, education, and much more that would otherwise simply not be available. And why? Because these are the basic values of Yoga itself—love, caring, mutuality, compassion, and well-being.

You can read more about the UN's Yoga Day Anniversary and some of these efforts in the free, beautifully illustrated, *Light on Light* e-magazine for the 2020 International Day of Yoga, its companion volumes for 2018-2022, and, for the 2020 International Day of Peace, the special issue entitled "Our Moment of Choice" (all at https://issuu.com/lightonlight). Let's choose the future we know is possible from our deepest senses of love and caring.

These are the heart of all our world's revered Wisdom Traditions and certainly the central message of Yoga.

- Enjoy the Related Practice: *Kriya for Awakening the Ten Bodies* [Yoga Practice Appendix 7 where I give an additional introduction to this Kriya]

INTERIOR AND EXTERIORS
– Balancing, with Nabhi Kriya with Prana and Apana
[Yoga Practice Appendix 8]

It does not take much looking around for any of us to realize our world has a problem with balancing, or even recognizing, interiors and exteriors.

In most situations today, when we go to work, we are expected to leave our interiors, our feelings, and life experiences at home. Even at home, members of families may simply ignore the upheavals or challenges that are going on in the interiors of their family members. Overall, we have little training or skills in this, either at work or at home.

The worlds of business, economics, and politics are nearly void of any recognition of interiors and the fact that they are a part, perhaps the major part, of what all human beings are. The result is, as the philosopher Ken Wilber says, business, economics, and politics are "flatlands" ruled by a shark tank mentality of competition, conflict, and the world of win/lose. Some of this is the heritage of 19th Century science that told us, in a misunderstanding of Charles Darwin's theories of evolution, that life is all about competition and survival of the fittest–one winning over the other–a world of I and Me, not We.

Today, as of 2015 or so, mainstream science has corrected this error of understanding, acknowledging that nature and evolution– particularly in species with intelligence and conscious choice– chose *neither* competition nor conflict but, instead, *cooperation*.

But, after 150 years of the myth of "Survival of the Fittest," it is a good question if this new understanding will quickly sink in. In fact, "Survival of the Fittest" is *true*, but the *definition* of fitness changes in complex systems and in intelligent species. It changes from competition to cooperation. You become more fit if you are a cooperator than if you are a competitor. This nuance was sadly missed by science for many decades but that's what new data now clearly shows.

Fortunately, science can quickly change its mind, and turn on its heels, when data changes (there are many examples). But there is no similar traction for a new idea, like cooperation, in arenas like politics, economics, and business where competition has always been the method and still remains the norm.

So, here enters the call of all practices and activities that acknowledge the interrelationship and "union" of interiors and exteriors, and Yoga (and Kundalini Yoga, in particular) is certainly major among these. It is likely that the depth to which we are "wired" for this kind of "union," the balance of the interior and exterior, is why Yoga has become so universally popular today. In fact, I'll bet you are thinking that it's quite nonsensical that this has been ignored for so long.

Even a quick look at the structure of Yogic practice—including silence, scripture, meditation, music, physical postures, and even dance—shows it is catering to this nurturing of both our exterior and our interior.

In fact, it is this discovery of, and balancing of, our interior and exterior life that is one part of the whole experience, as we have said, of "going down the rabbit hole," of immersing in the complex challenges of life and finding the answers and ways of life that really work for you.

The Chakras, the relationship of Kundalini practice to physiology and health, and the relationship of our individual humanity and the

Divine in Yogic Practice are all about this blending and balancing of interior life and exterior life.

In fact, it's safe to say that one of the reasons that this book exists, or that you've come to this book, is because, if you take a look, there is this challenge with recognizing and balancing the arenas of our exteriors and interiors. And, they are not even a binary reality—that is, they are not really separate as if you could walk from one to the other through a doorway. They are intricately and profoundly intertwined and interconnected, making the adventure quite an adventure after all.

- Enjoy the Related Practice: *Balancing, Nabhi Kriya with Prana and Apana* [Yoga Practice Appendix 8 where I give an additional introduction to these Practices]

HOW TO STAY NATURAL
– with Sat Kriya
[Yoga Practice Appendix 9]

Be curious—study, learn, see, travel—meet and greet new people and situations without judgment. Allow. That's a natural teaching.

On October 5th, 2018, a rare, very early, snowstorm changed the clime from a gorgeous summer day to sudden winter weather.

Instead of complaining, Awareness said, "Join the storm!" So, I got out the winter gear, jumped into the truck, and plowed through two feet of snow. I hit it hard—at first from my nervous energy—but then my inner climate control changed automatically, and I simply joined the storm, plowing the entire road. This in itself was a spontaneous awakening in awareness. I suddenly felt one with the entire winter season, which was announcing its presence with this unexpected snow. This gifted me for the rest of the winter, which was full of many more storms.

So... sometimes it's "off with the old" and "in with the new"—mentality and spiritually. This was a training opportunity—to join the storm without reacting, to act and not to react.

As I plowed, I realized this moment was an "off the mat" practice. Jump on the plow and meet the moment! With the challenge of going up the hill, pushing the heavy snow off to the side, backing up and repeating—each time, each series, was breaking down resistance or fear. It was a Kriya!

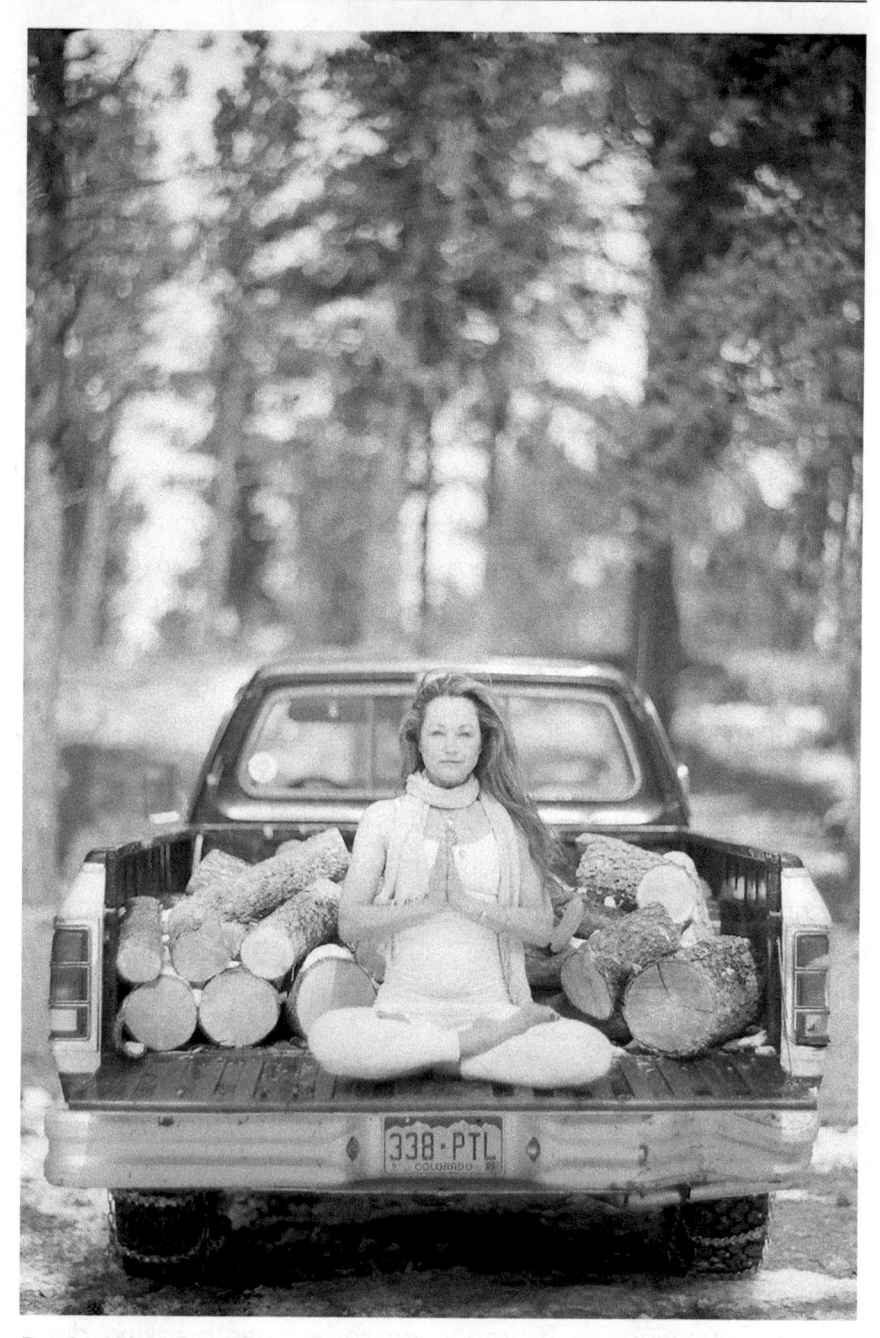

Rambo Kriya

The word comes from the Sanskrit root *"kri"* meaning "to do." With the suffix *ya*, as Kriya, it means action, deed, or effort. It's interesting that Kriya is derived from the same Sanskrit root as Karma!

This makes perfect sense since, in Yoga, Kriyas are series of postures (asanas), mudras, and music or sound. So, Kriya is often also defined as a series of actions aimed at achieving a certain result. That is certainly "natural." Think of any day-to-day series of actions you perform. Nearly all of them are to get a certain result: turn the lid of a jar with your hands to remove it; walk across the room to answer the door or the phone; or shut off the lights before going to bed. Pretty natural. If you didn't perform these actions in a certain sequence, they would simply not make sense.

You can *join* anything you are doing and experience it as a Kriya, instead of as a chore. I knew a lawyer who had learned this trick. He had to read through many boring files, but instead of moving through with drudgery, he would announce very loudly, as with the voice of a carnival barker, or comedian, "And the next file *is*!!!!"–and then he would laugh. Actually, everyone in his office got a bang out of it.

Becoming a Teacher has helped me to understand how to open this inner stage. Sometimes, as I progress through the stages of my life, it's like a trampoline–up and down, up and down–moving from one state of being to another.

No one is exempt from the basic needs of being here with a body and what is often called a "functional ego." Functional ego is different from ego-ego. You need to know your name; you need to sign your checks; someone needs to drive the car, etc.

When you mix it with the challenges of ego-ego, it can become quite complex–something we learn with time and maturity. When we find a mentor or teacher it's rather natural for us to put them on a pedestal. And then we'll notice their little traits that may be less pedestal-like. This will certainly be true of being in community with all of the followers of that teacher. You are all different personalities and likely on different paths. As the Dalai Lama says, you will always meet people who are on different paths. So, you will have your path; you'll be with a Teacher who has his or her path; and then there will be the Tribe around the Teacher as well. You'll need to get along with all of them, and they'll need to accept you too, just as you are. Each of you is on a journey.

This was certainly my experience. When I was in India and was given my spiritual name—Karuna—in Varanasi on the banks of the Ganga River, I really felt I didn't want to follow the practice that had led me to this ceremony. I wanted the ceremony, and to be in India, but I didn't identify with a lot of the details of the tradition going on around me. But, I knew that wherever you go with a group, there is a protocol. You have to follow what the group is doing, and the head Guru is "in charge," but at the same time, if you are attuned to a deeper sense of yourself or your destiny, all the parts might seem to not exactly fit together. When you're young and not clear of your path yet, such situations can be difficult.

But there is an essential stability that comes with just being natural about it—to navigate well in the context of "what is" when a bit of "what is" is coming from you and a bit from others. Having seen this pattern many times, I recommend a practice to balance the finding of your path called *Sat Kriya*. It helps you to be aligned, every day, with the intention to be strong and courageous and, in challenges, to be patient and tolerant. After all, there is a "Growing Up" part to every part of your "Waking Up," and to join this Waking Up and Growing Up, you need some "Cleaning Up." And, you need the Waking Up, the Growing Up, and the Cleaning Up if you're going to have the capability to be "Showing Up!"

Sat Kriya is a truly effective practice for Cleaning Up so that one can be Showing Up. It helps you to discern where you're at on your path, your levels of reactiveness and self-doubt. It is a very effective Kriya for clearing the subconscious of old patterns.

These patterns deserve attention in all of us. We want to establish new ways of being where we aren't meeting emotion with emotion, simply living in a ping-pong game of reactivity. Reactive patterns can be replaced with quiet and stability, and this is where the practice of "Rebirthing" comes in, and on a regular schedule. These practices go in and change the mindset. We actually change the mindset of the subconscious so that we are aware of what we are doing and are making skillful conscious choices, not just ones from habits that, through long durations, have become addictions.

I remember talking to many friends who have made this transition to a new stability. One of them said, "I remember the first time I truly realized I had a choice to do a certain behavior or not! It was amazing. There was enough spaciousness inside me that I could see, for the first time, that I was free to make a choice to do something, or not." For this person, it was a life-changer.

Actually, in such moments of freedom and epiphany, we become consciously aware of habits and how they are dominating our life. We can see them for ourselves and see that we are a step ahead. Then, as J. Krishnamurti said, we can finally get off that wheel of negative repetition.

We experience being the aware "Watcher." In that, we have the energy and capacity right there of Attention, and it's important to "catch it," to be fully aware. It may seem fleeting at first, coming and going, but in the consistency of routine that comes with the Yogic practice, the moments of clear seeing will return again and again—you'll clearly notice. So, we learn to pay attention and not to act and react in the same old way.

We have changed, and can change, the old reactive pattern. Understanding that Attention is timeless and that there are no competition-governed rewards or punishments, we feel that natural, innate freedom within us, and the old patterns simply slip away. I remember talking to a practitioner who had gone through this transition. Of some bad old habits she said, simply, "I stopped for a while, and then God just took it away."

One of the great gifts of the Sikh tradition is the understanding of the natural deity of the Presence of the Name—the Presence of God. In the ancient Sikh language called Gurmukhi, *Sat* means truth. *Nam* means name. Together, *Sat Nam* essentially translates into something deeper: "I am truth," or "Truth is my essence." This is one of the primal chants of Kundalini Yoga.

When one enters the *Gurdwara*, the holy space, the temple, one leaves weapons outside the door—not only symbolically, but one also naturally leaves behind one's animosity and judgment (you do not need them *there*) and bows at the feet of the Guru, or the teachings, of the wisdom, of the grace.

Here, things can happen which also teach us deep lessons, so I want to recount one that happened to me. There is a *seva* (an observance of service) called *Ishnon* which is cleaning the Gurdwara by rolling up all the rugs that are over the marble. One morning during summer solstice, I was rolling up the rugs in a playful way with one of my Sikh colleagues. We got it rolled up and were almost ready to pick it up and take it outside, when another Sikh brother came up and, being in a very different energy than me and my colleague, suddenly grabbed the carpet roll and jammed my finger between it and the heavy door. It so severely injured my right pinky that I needed medical attention.

This taught me that very odd things can occur in the natural space where people are just being exactly who they are. To me, it was a deep lesson in "Sat Nam." In the natural state, you've dropped any animosity or judgment. Everything needs to be attended to, and, that day, it seemed to include those varying energies bashing my finger between the Gurdwara carpets and the door. We took it all in stride and learned deeply from it.

Sat Nam! Truth is my identity, all of our identities, and that's how I choose to live. And I want to serve with delight, humor, mercy, forgiveness, compassion, and love. I want to polish my interior like the marble in a Gurdwara, and I want to live with all my beloveds with that kind of a humble heart.

- Enjoy the Related Practice: *Sat Kriya* [Yoga Practice Appendix 9 where I give an additional introduction to this Kriya]

GAUGING YOUR PROGRESS AND PREVENTING BURNOUT
– with Meditation Against Burnout
[Yoga Practice Appendix 10]

The Delight of the Frontier

By nature, being a pioneer means you're experiencing new things. This will be true of your Yogic experience because, likely, you've seen something in it you were attracted to and decided to try it. Sometimes, that can be a decision "from the head"—you "heard about it," or were looking around for something that could enhance your life and your health, and, obviously, Yoga was there on the shelf to be given a shot. Or, it could have been an experience more "from the Heart." You saw happiness, health, and well-being in people doing Yoga, and perhaps there was a moment when you said, "I want what that person has." Or, it could have even been more mystical where, when you observed the landscape of Yoga, there was something deep inside of you that spoke—one of those moments that "moved rivers within."

So, by nature, taking up Yoga practice will be the beginning of experiencing many things that are new. What is compelling about it is the opportunity to pick up the pieces of the Yoga landscape one by one, not only adding them to your toolkit but also experiencing the success and fulfillment of moving from one step to another. In Yoga, you might say each progression along the way is like a mini "hero's journey." The classic hero's journey, from the celebrated work of Joseph Campbell—author of *The Hero with a Thousand Faces*—is a journey from beginning to "muddle" (yes, muddle) and then resolution. Since Yogic practice is by nature a developmental one, moving step by step to higher and higher developmental levels, you will be finding the "beginning-muddle-resolution" pattern recurring again and again and again.

So, as a person initiating a serious Yogic path, it's good that we are aware of this recurrence of new situations from the beginning. We're prepared then to "be cool" about them, especially from what I've described earlier as the Neutral (Meditative) Mind. Being "cool" about them means being calm and patient, to always size up the attributes of what is going on (even feelings of "I've never seen this before!" or "Hum... what's going on here?" or even "This is weird!"). If you can cultivate that meditative place inside that gives you the space to step back a moment during your practice, you're not only going to be at a technical advantage for moving ahead step by step, but you're also actually already going to be cultivating "Watcher" consciousness. You'll realize there is no need to panic or feel the need to escape. There is no need to be reactive. Obviously, this is what good "free solo" climbers do as they inch their way up those precarious cliffs. They do exactly what the famous frontiersman whom I quoted earlier, Davy Crockett, said: at each step, "be sure you're right, then go ahead."

I mention this because such situations can be rather common in initial Yogic practice, and even in mature Yogic practice, because the practice itself is taking you from frontier to frontier. That's actually what frontier means—a place not seen before, at least by many. The words "frontier" and "pioneer" are connected in this way. And, for sure, Yogic practitioners are pioneers experiencing, what is for them, new frontiers.

LIGHT ON KUNDALINI

In the bigger view, this kind of awareness is often called "situational awareness." You've probably already intuited that this is what really good competitive athletes do—how they size up that "lane" leading to the basket or the goal line. What is going on here is that you are lending as many senses and viewpoints to your new experience as possible. You are gathering them all and seeing what the combinations tell you. This allows you to flow from frontier to frontier, often feeling, as you move from plateau to plateau and skill to skill, something like: "This may be new, but it sure feels *good*!" and, subsequently, "I'm *really* happy I discovered that." This is what it means when we say that no one really initiates you into your life as a Yogi; you initiate yourself. Another thing you'll discover, as a part of the community we have spoken of before, is that it's good and helpful to ask others what *they* are experiencing. You will get a lot of support in your own step by step journeys from hearing others remark: "Yes, that's exactly how I felt!" or "Yeah, me too; I didn't think I could do it, but shazam!" So, in Yogic practice, be aware that things and experiences can appear entirely new.

So, how often will this go on? Well, if you just page through a Yoga manual, and also realize that in Kundalini Yoga alone there are over four thousand formalized sequences (or Kriyas), you will learn that you have a lot of pioneering and frontier experiences to be had. It is likely that the initial weeks, months, and years of what will be the entry into your life-practice will be one delightful frontier after another.

Mid-Passage

So, let's jump ahead. Let's jump ahead not only regarding your experience of Yogic practice but also to the changes that your body, and your emotional makeup, will go through, especially as you naturally age. When you are a few weeks, months, or years into your practice you are going to have seen, and deeply appreciate, how the structure of building your Yoga practice, step by step, has helped you to gauge your progress. You may also notice that something that had been lacking in your life experience before Yoga was that, previously, you never had a sense of how to be aware of, gauge, or measure your life's progress. This makes sense especially if you think that the life of your Yogic practice is actually about just getting "better and better," "healthier and healthier," and "happier and happier." But it's important to realize that one of the things that will *also* be new are natural challenges that simply come with time.

On the one hand, to everything in life there is a transition from the "Disneyland" or "Honeymoon" experience into "mid-Passage" or where, for our human makeup, sometimes "familiarity can even breed contempt," where things can "wear out" or no longer hold the charm they once did. Also, there are changes that will occur with just the natural aging of our bodies *and* our life-experience. It appears there is a "mid-life crisis" natural to every human endeavor. The definition of "mid-Passage" in psychological terms says it all: "mid-Passage begins when a person is obliged to ask *anew* the question of meaning, which once enlivened the younger person's imagination, but had then been effaced over the years." Note that the definition uses the word "obliged." In other words, it is likely it will happen to everyone.

The important thing here is knowing that that, too, is natural. You will inevitably find those moments where you ask yourself things such as: "I can't just keep looking back to when I was twenty; how can I feel good *now*?" or "Instead of looking back to when I was in a relationship, what is the healthiest way for me to be me *now*? or "How can I move into a new career instead of looking back at the one, two, or three I have already had?"

With your body, you also will likely have to scale down, addressing questions such as: "How should my diet be different now that I'm getting older?" or "How has the long, pounding run I used to take become the mindful walk that works for me now, years later?" Believe me, you will feel completely in sync with this process of gauging yourself once you realize that patterns *now* have to be different than patterns *then*—and that you've found the new pattern that is just perfect for who you are now. Your patterns are different now; your hormones and physiology are different now; and your visions forward and in rear-view are also different. Everything has changed. So, what skills can be learned for gauging our progress and our progressions? This is part of the journey.

What about Burnout?

"Burnout" has to be one of the most idiosyncratic and individualistic phenomena on the planet. Some people seem inexplicably immune to it—it will never happen. Yet, even the best of others can run into a snag and suddenly find things topsy turvy. For deeply spiritual people, sometimes burnout creeps in because, from time to time, we somehow forget the bottom-line truths of our Conscious lives, our potentials, our birthright. This can simply inadvertently happen in all of our doing-doing-doing. I think sometimes, in all of the rushing and doing, we inadvertently revert back to a less conscious mind, and old mental patterns deeply ingrained in us sneak in again. I liken it to when we're driving along in a car and find ourselves veering off toward the edge, and we suddenly, rather automatically, "self-correct" with the steering wheel.

When those moments occur in the lives of the best of us, we need to do something similar—just stop for a moment and remind ourselves of who we are and what this Divine life is about. We need to remind ourselves of the great truths of Awakened consciousness—that the path *is* the destination, and that we have been there all the time, even in shadowed moments.

Sometimes, that moment of reassessment is all we need. The simple reminder of that truth helps us to get out of the false stories that have enveloped us—what one poet called "our false disasters." As I said in my chapter about Healing Grief, some 95% of suffering comes from our stories of "who did what to whom," and this kind of suffering from "he said/ she said" is not the same as the real suffering from grief of tragic loss that causes a real energy disruption in our system. It has that effect on us only if we let emotion and commotion do that. Taking that moment to remind ourselves of the great Truths, tuning into something beautiful, calming, or inspiring, we can usually readily find relief. Sometimes, we can even have a good laugh at ourselves.

But, other times, our need for recuperation may be more severe, and this is where attention to it with Yoga practice can, with surety, come to our aid.

A great practice for this kind of remembrance and perspective, and attention to the need for real recuperation, is the Meditation Against Burnout. Like the steps in Healing Grief, the structure of the meditation with the related asanas and mudras is designed to calm the body first, to create the meditative neutral energy flow and allow the wisdom of the True Self to naturally come back to the body's temple. I am sure you will find this meditation always useful, and successful, in those moments when things have simply been too much. So, it's good that we cap this section with a practice that, again, brings us back from zero point to rebirth—that "way out" of the rabbit hole that I promised you is always there, a way through every block.

- Enjoy the Related Practice: *Meditation Against Burnout* [Yoga Practice Appendix 10 where I give an additional introduction to this Meditation]

GRACE AND GRACEFULNESS IN TRANSITIONS
– with Nahbi Kriya
[Yoga Practice Appendix 11]

A Flood of "Fierce Grace"

All was going so well. I was even pinching myself as I was driving up the road to my beautiful mountain home in the high country above Boulder, Colorado (see https://issuu.com/lightonlight/docs/lightonlight_issue_1, p. 45-51). My son had been visiting me from London with his newlywed, and they were moving to San Francisco. They had even decided to stay an extra few days, so their stuff was piled in the hallway ready for their eventual trip west. So, we would have extra time to enjoy each other, sit by the fire, and drink in the view of the mountain peaks that form the horizon along my back deck. These two weeks together were such a precious time. I had even told a friend that, after their visit, it was going to feel strange going back to an empty house.

In due course, I was seeing them off to California and, alone again, was weaving myself back up my mountain road, first from pavement and then to gravel. In stark contrast to the sunny days while my son and new daughter-in-law had been with me, it was now starting to rain. It seemed almost fitting as an end to what had been such a wonderful time. But as I came around my greenhouse and shed, to pull into the driveway where I would normally be

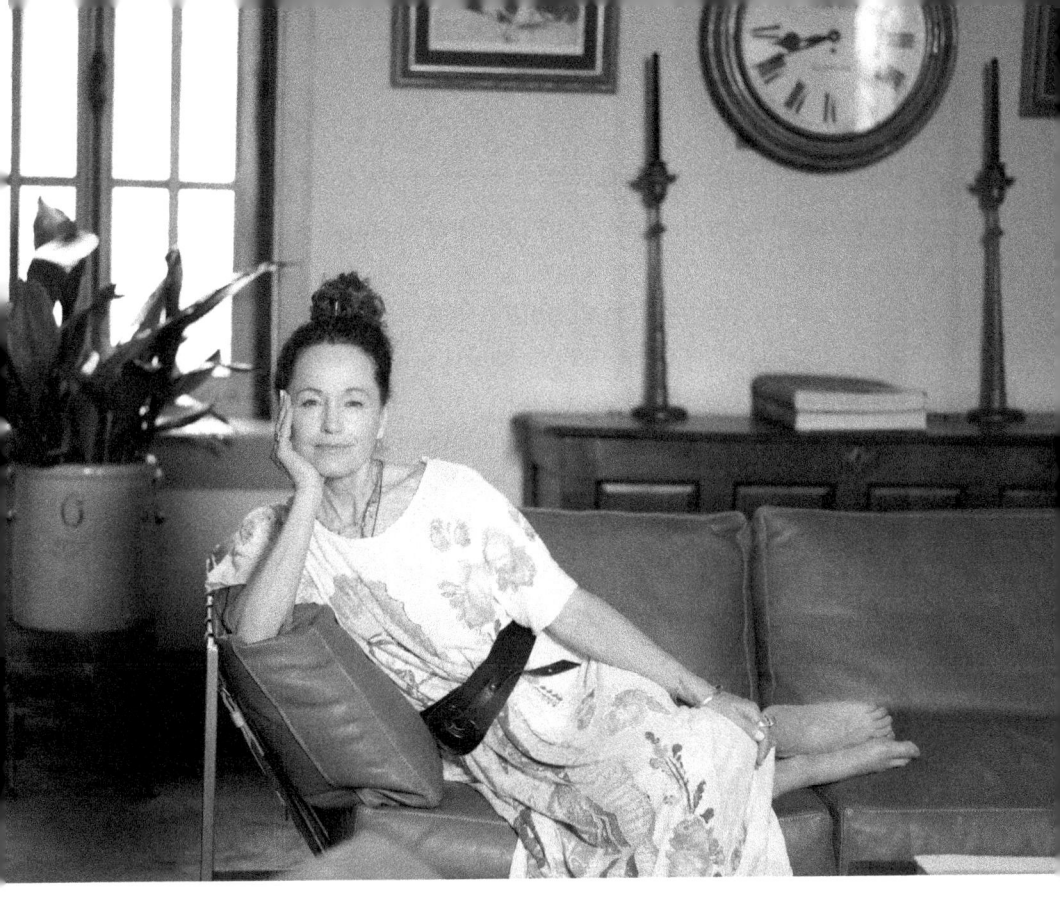

Love Unconditionally

greeted by the bright blue window boxes that frame the windows of my house, something both strange and incomprehensible took my sight. Oddly enough, it was Halloween, and, as if from a Halloween movie, all of the windows of my house were frosted over *from within*. It was the strangest thing I had ever seen, and I immediately knew something extremely odd, or even terrible, must have happened.

Of course, I immediately ran to the front door, which would usually open into my large, windowed, greeting room. I was on alert—but not prepared for what I would see. Torrents of water were running and spraying down from all the levels of my house as if in a violent, interior rainstorm. I stood there in shock. Wow, was this actually happening? I had never seen anything like this in my life.

Then it hit me that I had better move fast and figure out what to do first. That moment was like a sudden slideshow flashing through both my mind and mind's eye—gifted (I realize now!) by everything I had learned from my years of devoted Yoga practice—*stability*, *alertness*, and *calm*. So, instead of paying attention to my *immediate* human emotions, which were telling me to yell, shout, cry out, or just run around, I was able to become very calm and simply ask myself, "OK, how do I react *usefully*?"

The phone was working, so I called a neighbor who I thought might know what was behind all this. They told me to immediately shut off my well, since it was likely that something might have gone horribly wrong with the water system. I did that and *then* immediately called my insurance company. I figured they would have a "bead" on what was going on and could advise me on what to do next, since—first off—it was going to take at least a half hour for anyone to reach my home. Secondly, they would know, from my policies, what was relevant here. Wonderfully, they were immediately friendly and cooperative and dispatched someone, right away, toward my home.

It was then that it hit me that I could take a deep breath and absorb what had just been happening. I stood still awhile and looked around at everything with a bit of wonderment. Of course, the inevitable question then came across my mind: "Why did this happen?"

I suppose this is the question that nearly everyone would ask in this kind of sudden, seemingly inexplicable, disaster. So, it was *my turn*, and these were the thoughts that bubbled around in me for the near hour it took for the insurance personnel to arrive. Immediately, relief came with the first "prompt" they gave to me after looking around. I had done nothing wrong; it was not my fault; and my insurance would cover *all* of what appeared to be quite a major disaster.

But, as you know, this is not the end of how we mortals question why something happened. And, here, some deep spiritual searching, and questions and answers, are relevant to *us all*. So, let's explore it.

Like you, I could not quit asking myself about *why* this had happened—especially on the heels of such a wonderful set of days with my family in my lovely home—a house which, in nearly thirty years, had not endured any major disruption or damage at all (except once an incursion of bees). Had I done something wrong? Was this because I hadn't done "this" or "that"? Was this "pay back" for God knows what? I must say that, especially in the context of Yoga practice, and our sometimes less than mature or well-educated understandings of "Karma" (cause and effect), these are the array of questions that would occur to any of us about what was going on here.

I must *also* say that I'm not one to immediately "go with" some abstract notion of cause and effect, especially ones that infer "blame" on the victim! There are plenty of easily induced notions of abstract powers and energies, rewards, and punishments: "Was the Feng Shui off? Had my house been crying out for help, and I had not listened? Was there some distant and unrelated thing that I had done, and this was my punishment?"

The deep problem with such notions is that they often end up blaming the *victim*—which, in this case, was *me*. Further, it's just as likely in life that things can happen rather at random, with no actual "real reason" at all. I think if we are healthy people, our worldview on these matters lands somewhere in between. Of course, there *are* spiritual reasons that things happen. But there are also things that "just happen." Wisdom appears somewhere in between. I remember when His Holiness the Dalai Lama commented on someone's suggesting that the Indonesian Tsunami happened because of the collective karma of the people in the region. He said that, abstractly, that might be true *but* that the matters involved were by nature so complicated one would be "a fool" (he said) to outrightly suggest such a cause—especially to the media.

The Lesson

Well, without my knowing it, there was a big surprise in store for me in learning from this "disaster" that had just unfolded in my life. And, that is why I'm writing about it.

How to even say it? From the fierce, yet amazingly bountiful, Grace of this experience, I not only got my "doctor's degree" in rejecting the tendency to play the "analysis game," the "why game," or the "blame game," but I was *also* to be shown something I really think I had not seen before. And *that kind of thing* is a surprise for any of us!

You know, I have been so lucky to live the last decades of my life tied up within our world's "spiritual community." Here, I get to work with such wonderful people in the context of such beautiful worldviews *and* lifestyles about love, mutuality, reciprocity, kindness, compassion, and on and on. To be honest, I think, over the years, I got used to thinking that it was these *contexts* that made these people and the way they lived so special. After all, I was also a *teacher*. So—actually—I was spending my life "teaching *others*" about these ways of life—about love, mutuality, reciprocity, kindness, compassion, and so on. I had "my own loop" in which all these wonderful things happened regularly for me.

So, you can imagine me really being both side-swiped and flabbergasted when—thrown out of my element, thrown out of my home, thrown out of my teaching center, and just thrown out on the world—suddenly, *here*, among all these "strangers" were all these wonderful people running to help me (out of *real* authenticity and *real* concern, offering help and assistance from the biggest to the smallest) and yet not claiming, or even referencing, any kind of "spiritual" reason for their goodness or good deeds, or some "spiritual practice" they had immersed in to make them so giving and so caring.

Let me just say it again. Here was this amazing rush of people, full of love, care, compassion, and a desire to help, *irrespective* of background or belief, or even any stated identification with "people of Spirit, or Faith, or Spiritual Practice," or anything even close to it!

What We Don't Hear Enough About

We all hear these stories about "when people come together" in a crisis or after a sudden disaster, but I honestly think we don't hear *enough* of it. I don't think we've plumbed to the required depth what the real lesson is here. There is something we learn about in these times which is the thing we really should be reaching for *all the time*—because it's *there*, in our *nature*. We need to reach for how that nature in us can be acting all the time, not just when a crisis brings us together.

This is not something new. You've heard this before. It's nearly a cliché. But think about it—this was exactly what was happening to me in "my disaster." It was reminding me of something that had, like for all of us, become a bit masked or even perhaps forgotten. Is that why we need these reminders?

In this disaster in my life, from which people could have just walked away or done what was the "token" required by their job or profession, I was gifted a steady flow of caring and help from countless people who came into this predicament from every angle—from the details of insurance, the arrangements for temporary and then long-term accommodation, and the meeting of immediate personal disaster needs (as all of my belongings were either destroyed or removed and sequestered) to the plans and planning for restoring and rebuilding (if possible at all).

I had come to expect this kind of behavior (and teach it too) from people of "spiritual practice, ethics, and ideals," but I was overwhelmed by these unbelievable people—on this planet earth—who never even heard of Yoga or this or that spirituality or religion, who knew nothing about me or my past, or who never voiced an opinion about *me*. As all this was occurring before me, it seemed like just one *natural* spiritual practice or "a practice with Spirit" as I soon came to tag it.

Rebuilding

In the subsequent time when, suddenly homeless, I was first living in a hotel, and then a "temporary" house, I knew I was processing through something "big" for me. I was operating completely outside my old element, going to courses, classes, and associations I had never even heard of before simply "because they were what's around" and knowing, all the time, that I was in the learning process about this lesson: "You're healthy. You can do this. You can trust this. This is not something you would have designed for yourself, but it was apparently designed for *you*."

It was not clear how many of the precious personal things I had accumulated in my home for decades were recoverable or restorable from all that was taken out and sequestered. I was amazed, however, as I have mentioned above, that even the technicians discussing with me what could be saved, and how, seemed to be as devoted as I was to some kind of "happy ending" if at all possible. Of course, you can say, "Well, you were paying them!"

but I can assure you it was deeper than that. And, I was legitimately proud of myself when I slept well at night in those "strange" and "unfamiliar places."

It occurred to me that for all the "rebirthing classes" that I offered out of the Yoga studio that was part of my home for 27 years, I seemed to have been offered the biggest "rebirthing" of my own! That in itself was an experience—standing in the Yoga studio I put together, floored, and furnished over years of dedication—seeing it all in front of me, in a *heap*!

I—the person who was always helping others—learned what it meant to accept help *from* others, and the amazement I experienced in how freely that help was offered and given was what really emblazoned the lesson here. Standing in my temporary house, I was able to honestly say to myself, "If there are any such things, *this* was a meant to be."

So, when Denise Scotto (Chair of the International Day of Yoga Committee at the United Nations) with whom I've worked regularly as Host Editor of *Light on Light Magazine* for the annual special issues on the International Day of Yoga asked me to write about "how I survived all this," I realized there really *was* something to say, and a *lesson* to report about.

- https://issuu.com/lightonlight/docs/lightonlight_un_idy
- https://issuu.com/lightonlight/docs/lightonlight_un_idy_2019

There is part of the Yoga Sutras that talks about "stealing"—the taking advantage of abundance and then the hidden grace of our big falls *down* and "back to zero." It appears that Source knows the ones who can be taken back to zero, and when. Certainly, when one sees a home of nearly three decades reduced to a shell full of dust, one knows one has been offered a zero point. *And*, that it's time to rebuild—everything.

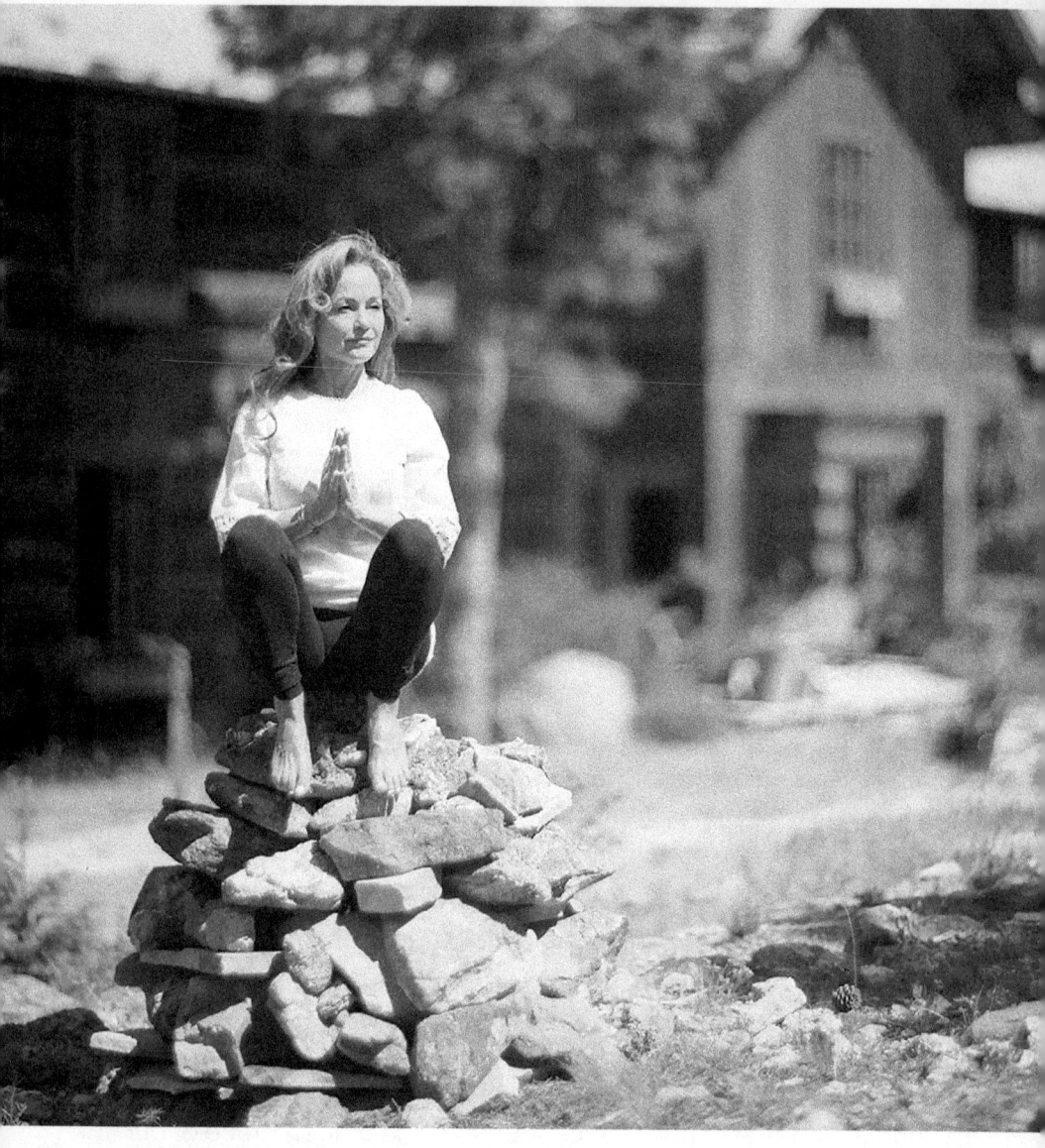

Rebirth

- Enjoy the Related Practice: *Nahbi Kriya* [Yoga Practice Appendix 11, where I give an additional introduction to this Kriya]

MORE ON YOGIC LIFE

Having just finished an Inspiration and Practice on "Gauging Your Progress," let's do exactly that. At this point in the adventure of this book, you've journeyed from Invitation to Introduction, and then on to Information and Inspiration. We just combined Inspiration with eight specific experiential Yoga practices so you could experience firsthand how Yoga practice and real life are truly one.

Now, I want to share more and more about Yoga—and Yogic life—across the truly opulent landscapes of:

- meditation, mantra, and music,
- special practices for nurturing your unfolding yogic journey, and
- yogic health, wellness, and fitness.

Yoga and Sound – Meditation, Mantra, and Music

Yoga and sound are inseparable. In the chapter "Yoga Cosmology," you'll remember my description "Yoga and the Structure of Everything." Therein, from the largest to the smallest, all things are made up of intertwinements of the same thing—all a vast multiplicity of appearances, all made of the same Substance of Divine Nature.

One of the deepest realizations of Awakening is "everything is the same—made of the same stuff—and it's all Divine." This is what led the ancients to declare: "As above, so below."

Yoga cosmology begins with the primal "Name" or "Sound," of and from which All is comprised and unfolds. A sound uttered as "*Om*" or "*Aum*" is not only seen as the primal, originating, vibration but the familiar Sanskrit representation for *Om* or *Aum* is also the symbol of the Wisdom Traditions of the Indian subcontinent, and their offspring. Precise meanings, and broader implications, concerning Om and Aum then richly unfold across the millennial narratives of Buddhism, Hinduism, Sikh & Santism, Jainism, and more. The universe is experienced as vibrational—the elements of vibration being the *"nada"* of which all things are made, from the most primal, originative, all-embracing of sounds (like *Om, Aum*) to the multiplicities (even cacophonies) of nature, to ultimately "the music of the cosmos" and the Divine itself. Silence is seen as alive with *nada*, full of meanings and messages, and the "divine music" is seen as reaching from the deepest of within to the vastness of with-out. Inherently living in such a cosmology, all the Yogas are often called *"Naad"* or "Naad Yogas," that is, born of the all-encompassing sound that includes both the Ultimate Divine and our own human aspect as divinity. It should not surprise us then that modern science also has come to speak of our cosmology and cosmic origins in terms of sound—"string theory" and the "big bang." We can assume rightly that as science continues to elaborate the elegance of this cosmos in which we find ourselves, it will turn even more to words that reflect or imply sound—and music.

Meditation

With a mind to understanding even silence as alive with *nada*—carrying meanings and messages—let's now explore, and further unwrap, "Meditation." Then we'll move from there to Mantra and Music, all appearances within the intertwined realms of *naad*-vibration. Before thinking of it as part of the realms of vibration, you may have greeted this subtitle "Meditation" with a sigh. It's a huge topic.

Meditation is a word very difficult to define, as it characterizes pursuits of religions, spirituality, and reflection across the world for millennia. Along with mantra, across the world's written languages, the oldest records specifically referring to meditation are found in the scriptures (the *Vedas*) of the Wisdom Traditions of the Indian subcontinent—from some 5,000 years ago. They are reported in oral traditions for at least 5,000 years before that. But this can be misleading, suggesting perhaps a purely Eastern origin of "meditation"—and then its coming to the West. The West already had its own traditions of meditation in Christianity, the Sufism of Islam, Judaism, and across the polytheisms of Greece and Rome. The Greeks called it "*melete*" (mental exercise), and the Roman thinker Plotinus actually taught methods of meditation in the 3rd Century CE. These words, attributed to Plotinus, might well be those of an Eastern Sage or Yoga Master:

> "If you imagine you're different from the all-pervading Divine Being, you are not yet in the fully illumined state. When you and it are perfectly one, with no sense of even the possibility that you could be two, then you have attained real understanding and a true perception of your highest self, the true inner being which never departs from complete perfection."

In the Latin of Plotinus, the word for meditation, *meditatio*, or as a verb, *meditari*, meant to think, devise, ponder, or contemplate—quite a range of endeavors! English readily adopted its word—meditation—from that Latin origin, undoubtedly through the historical influence of the Roman Catholic Church. Whatever the history, today we universally recognize that activities associated with meditation significantly relieve worry, anxiety, stress, depression, and pain. Not only does meditation ease these maladies, but it also enhances positive attributes of well-being like self-esteem, peacefulness, and clear thinking. Today, research goes on around the world concerning the positive effects of meditation on physical, mental, and spiritual health.

Given this universality, it is no surprise that meditation has been a foundational part of Yoga from its beginning, and no accident that meditation naturally companions all the other aspects of Yoga.

One could actually suggest that meditation is even more than "foundational" in Yoga, is actually the ultimate itself–the silence, the listening Presence, in which all of the other attributes of Yoga ultimately find their home. It is here that the "Awakening" emerges and abides–called by so many names across all the traditions–*moksha*, *vimukti*, *kaivalya*, *samadhi*, *nirvana*, the Divine Union, nondual consciousness, etc. Different words for this ultimate state occur in over one hundred languages, and meditation is its pursuit, its invitation, its enticement.

Understanding meditation in its biggest sense, as both journey and destination, requires universal and historic understanding of its roots in who we are. From the time our human ancestors first shared moments of quiet with beloveds, or pondered the stars, or built ancient monuments (like Stonehenge in England, Kokino in Macedonia, Taosi in China, and so many others) to track and embrace the seasons, *meditatio*–meditation, quiet, presence–has been a part of our nature, our beacon for "going Home."

It is no surprise then that in Yoga it is the final limb of the Eight Limbs of Patanjali, the eight limbs that lead to that ultimate *moksha*, *vimukti*, *kaivalya*, *samadhi*, *nirvana*, the Divine Union, or nondual consciousness. You have the ethical disciplines (*yamas*), the cautions (*niyamas*), the body postures (*asanas*), the breathwork (*pranayama*), the mastery of the senses (*pratyahara*), the focus on the Divine (*dharana*), the employment of meditation (*dhyana*), and, finally, the Ultimate coming home (by whatever name). Thus, certainly, the "deep dive" of Kundalini Yoga, with its focus on the mystical–the foundational–attention to meditation is paramount.

Sharings

I cannot think or talk about meditation without remembering the counsel I, and so many others, so fortunately received from our beloved fellow-Coloradoan friend Fr. Thomas Keating. Fr. Keating, known to his friends as "Fr. Thomas," is, of course, the renowned Trappist monk, interfaith leader, and founder of Centering Prayer, Contemplative Outreach, and the decades long Snowmass Interreligious Dialogues. From the latter were published the "Nine Points of Agreement Among the World's Religions" in the book, *The Common Heart*, by Fr. Thomas, and others, in 2006.

I was able to visit with him numerous times, with interfaith friends and even with my family. Since we all shared this background of the pursuit of all the world's traditions of ultimate potential and birthright of "Awakening," we often talked of the "nondual." As all of us knew, this was a word that today is quite well understood in both the world's spiritual traditions and in modern psychology and consciousness studies. But a decade or more ago, the commonality of the Awakening experience across all the world's traditions was much less known. Persons like Fr. Keating, and his colleague (and friend-of-my-friend Dr. Kurt Johnson), Br. Wayne Teasdale, were part of nurturing what became the eventual melding of this global understanding, first through the Monastic Interreligious Dialogue which "back then" often communicated through mimeograph machines, long before word processing and computers became common.

Little by little, the understanding of the birthright of Awakening—as it is called in the Kundalini Yoga tradition—became more and more well known, capped by hundreds of books worldwide, among them being *The Common Heart* and Teasdale's *The Mystic Heart: Discovering a Universal Spirituality in the World's Religions*, both considered classics today. So, working in the context of this heritage and the interspiritual landscape further embraced in Kurt

Johnson's *The Coming Interspiritual Age*, Adam Bucko and Rory McEntee's *The New Monasticism*, Mirabai Starr's *God of Love*, Will Keepin's *Belonging to God*, and so many others, it has been a privilege indeed. We have spent many wonderful hours together, along with some of the great contemporary teachers of nonduality like Pamela Wilson, Annette Knopp, Loch Kelly, and Rupert Spira.

Fr. Keating, always jovial at best and, of course, always deep, used to quip about "how far we can go with this *nonduality*," and then he would chuckle. I have always remembered Fr. Keating's differentiation of "meditation" and "contemplation." The latter is a word more common to Christianity, but I want to share Fr. Thomas' take on it. Fr. Keating likened meditation to an inquiry, an asking, a seeking, an investigating. But then he would say, "When someone answers your inquiry, your asking, your seeking, it becomes a dialogue, and that is contemplation."

Hearing that from Fr. Thomas, I could not help but remember the instances in my own life, and I have mentioned so many herein, where when I reached out, I got an answer—even if it did not come right away. I can trace those moments from that time I was sitting in the hotel room in Paris wondering where my life-path was taking me, to my first meetings with Yoga and responding to that calling, to the entreaty by my mentor for me to become a Teacher. We come to realize in Yoga, and especially Kundalini Yoga, the adventure of the "deep dive" we have committed to. In it, we find all the paradoxes, all the twists, turns, and nuances that the Great Mystics speak of. And we find, and I know you will too, that moment—or moments—when we are on the other side, at the destination, but may not quite know how we got there. I think of this now in writing this part of this book, recalling the month-long time I spent talking with Kurt Johnson before the memorial and tribute event held for Fr. Thomas in Aspen and Snowmass (July 13-14, 2019). We finished some three hundred pages of notes for this book before driving over to attend that remembrance event.

Mantra

Like meditation, the history of mantra is both ancient and mysterious. Our common English usage from the original Sanskrit—Mantra—has diverse meanings, and its origins are shrouded in millennia of history. Its most basic meaning—as some form of "chant" either with or without musical context—places it in virtually every spiritual tradition around the world. At deepest depth, it reflects the understanding across our world's spiritual traditions that sound is fundamental, if not the very origination, of existence itself. Accordingly, our understanding of mantra stems all the way from these deepest meanings across our world's spiritual traditions to modern colloquial usages in sport, politics, and even advertising! We sometimes don't realize that all this modern activity is mantra as well!

All of these contexts acknowledge the power of such utterance—that is, what is called "numinous sound." Numinous means that it evokes powerful action and reaction. From this has come the common understanding—from religion to fantasy fiction—that mantra, or chant, has magical or spiritual power. Looking at mantra's deepest historical roots, we learn much by considering what the word is taken to mean across multiple languages and traditions—including "true words," "sacred utterance," "divine words," and even "secret words."

Mantra is at least 3,500 years old as recorded in our world's religious texts. If we readily assume it was part of other early cultures for which we have no direct written proof, this pushes it back 7-10,000 years. Assuming it also was naturally a part of eon's-past indigenous cultures, this dates it back beyond 50,000 years. In fact, scientists debate whether mantra and chant might have pre-dated language, or even been a precursor to language, given its obvious association in ancient indigenous cultures, and even early species of humans, with rhythm, action, dance, and the like. Early cave paintings portray dance and celebration, and we must assume it was accompanied by some kind of collective rhythmic activity. When such cave paintings show drums, we know this for certain.

Along the historical timeline of Yoga I shared earlier in this book, mantra became first prominent in the Vedic Period (2000-1000 BCE). It had further resurgence during the more current Bhakti Period (1470-1710 CE) because of its evocative devotional power. Writings of these eras contain over 10,000 varieties of mantra. The renaissance of mantra in the Bhakti Period, just over four centuries ago, obviously bridged it powerfully into the Yoga practices that we know today.

I'm going to spend some time on this because exploring and sharing the gifts and mysteries of mantra is personally important to me. It was not only my own entry point into Yogic life, but I also have since spent years supporting, sponsoring, and producing Yogic music and activities all around the world. And I will say much more about that—fondly—a bit later.

The Deep Mysteries of Mantra

From the varieties of mantra, and their reaching back some 4,000 years, we learn some important things about the nature of mantra itself—what it is and why it is so evocative. We learn something about both our Divine and human natures when we look at the emotional, psychological, and spiritual power of combined recitation, call and response, music, and movement. Modern neuroscience understands how our brains emit stimulating, even arousing, natural chemicals when basic body motions are combined with forms of recitation, call and response, chant, or music. On the happy side, people often comment not only on how relaxing and calming sound—especially music—can be, but also on how, when they hear music, their bodies often simply just want to move. On the less happy side, we also witness the angry and violent vibrations that can be stirred up by unscrupulous politicians, agitators, or "rabble-rousers" who use the same means to fire up a crowd. So, without a doubt, the spiritual and physical ingredients in what underlies mantra are powerful.

Some of the intriguing elements concerning mantra are obvious once mentioned, but otherwise, are perhaps simply not thought of. They include these fascinating aspects, and we need to look at each.

- Why do some mantras have literal meanings and some do not?
- Why can mantras be both personal and communal?
- Do mantras "carry" spiritual energies or "powers" from their spiritual traditions?

Meaning and Mantra

Some mantras have literal meaning, and some do not. This fact has both historical and functional significance. Perhaps you have forgotten, but the same is true in modern music. Modern vocal music contains literal words, of course, but also utterances without meaning. Yet, those utterances are as important to the character, appeal, and power of the music as are the words with meaning. We see this in the recurrent role and relationship of the "lead" and "backup" singers. Technically, these words without literal meaning are called "background runs and riffs" and are usually added by background singers but are sometimes also "sung" by the lead singer. Examples are myriad, but I'll list two you'll recognize right away: James Taylor, singing as lead, "Come-a, come-a, come-a, come-a, come, come, Yeah, yeah, yeah," and Manfred Mann's quirky, "Do wah diddy diddy dum diddy do." There are countless other examples from backup singers. If you jump online and "google" famous backup singing lines, you'll find familiar ones like "doo-wop-dowah," "shoo wapp," "do lah," "oh lati da," and even "beep, beep, beep, beep, yeah" (that one's from the Beatles' "Drive my Car"). An entire music genre based on words without specific meanings is thus aptly called "Doo Wop."

To musicologists and anthropologists, the message is simple: moving rhythmic utterance from what modern music calls "riffs," "runs," or "nonsense lyrics" is actually built in to what we humans are wired for, and music would not be music without it. This brings special meaning to our understanding that what has become "mantra" in Yoga shares this mixture of specifically meaningful words and just rhythmic utterances. This recognition brings up another question about mantra—when does it involve music and when not, and how did that come about? Let's look further into that.

Looking across the shrouded history of our world's religions, we see a long history of communal activity called "recitation," that is, call and response. This was of obvious communal value for bonding and recognition. This fascinates scientists because science actually suggests that mantra is what birds do with birdsongs! They are fundamental communication but most often not decipherable into precise meanings!

With this mysterious background of mantra, most historians agree that our human development of music, mantra, movement, ritual, and their interrelationships was likely a rather meandering historical process appearing variously across myriad cultures. Of course, we *do* know that much ancient sharing of the narratives and stories by our earliest human cultures came from the passing down of oral (that is, sound-related) instruction, long before languages were written down. Thus, historians debate which came first—ritual, mantra, music, or specific language? We think we can guess that these elements were always intertwined, simply because they are that way today in our own experience. As they likely did, today, we still mix recitation, call and response, mantra, music, movement, and ritual. This helps us to understand how ancient the methods of Yoga actually are.

So, when were the varieties of musical instruments added, and synchronous movement? What are the origins of what has now become globally known, and celebrated, as "Kirtan" (about which I will write much more separately below)? Obviously, it began with drums, whose usage in religious ceremony is as old as depicted in cave paintings known to be 17,000 years old! First drums, of course, and then all varieties of sound producing instruments were added, culture to culture. If we look back into history, we see, across the religions embracing Yoga, a movement from recitation and chant without any musical context to the adding of music for both recitation and chant, and call and response, and, ultimately, the addition of more and more musical instruments. Within communities and their histories of sacred music evolved antiphons (musical bookends starting and ending community gatherings), hymns (devotional songs), and, finally, more intricate compositions that carried far more complex sacred narratives and stories. In most cultures, these became permanent fixtures, century to century in their lexicons of sacred expression, and then, especially meaningful to the cohesion of spiritual community culture, choreographed recitation, music, and movement. And that became religious ritual–powerful and transformative then, and powerful and transformative today.

Mantra, Personal and Communal

You'll remember one of the initial definitions of mantra that I previously gave–"secretive words." Thus, in so many traditions, there is the custom of personalized mantra, that is, the mantra given from a teacher to a follower to aid their path. Private mantra in this sense, as "revealed" to the individual person, parallels the role that mantra always played as a part of oral, and later written, traditions–being seen as "revealed Truth." The use of personal mantra is also deeply tied to our understandings of the esoteric power of mantra which I will tell you much more about below, and the same esoteric powers apply to collective use of mantra as well.

Historically, Yoga traditions have varied on the role of mantra as personal (even secret) or collective. The tradition of my own training, the Sikh tradition, was among the first to stress the collective, community role of mantra, celebrated together in the sacred spiritual gathering places (or "Gurdwaras") of that tradition. Both private and collective mantra are important elements in Kundalini Yoga's special attention to the practice called *"Sadhana."* Sadhana (the same in Sanskrit and as Anglicized) is the most special private *and* collective gathering, tailored daily by the Kundalini Yoga community, to nurture the ongoing development of its followers and adepts. These are people much like yourself, developing your yogic path, even as you read this book. Sadhana truly creates a mystical nest—a landing zone—into which can drop Divine soul inspirations, discernments, and determinations, all facilitating the forward movement of your path, step by step. Sadhana is so important that I later devote an entire chapter to it.

Yoga (or something much like it), across our world's rich Wisdom Traditions, plays a principal role in the intertwining of worship, meditation, mantra, music, movement, ritual, and the larger cultural narrative. Yoga or Yoga-like practices are well known in Hinduism, Buddhism, Jainism, and Sikhism. If we look to traditions that simply don't use the word "Yoga" (or a word close to it), we find Yoga-like practices also in Zoroastrianism, Taoism, Shinto, and also Christianity (for example, with the Shakers and in modern Centering Prayer). In my chapter on Ayurveda, I will review many of these similar practices. Across all these traditions, the varieties noted above of sounds, words, movement, and rituals all pertain. And mantras, of course, can even be repeated silently in the mind. In Yoga Practice, our repertoire of such activities will mostly likely derive from the cultural tradition in which we are practicing. Particularly in today's global interfaith and interspiritual contexts, there is already tremendous interrelating and intermixing of the practices available from across the traditional and cultural schools of Yoga.

Here, one historic distinction is important. Kundalini Yoga, as it comes most explicitly from the Sikh tradition, has always been a more public and collective culture with regard to music and mantra. Some of this results from the multifaith roots of Sikhism as it arose on the Indian subcontinent but, in any event, Sikhism is one of the first historical traditions wherein mantras are considered public and are open for everyone to use. I will share about this more in my later chapters on "Community" and *seva* (selfless service).

The Esoteric Power of Mantra

We know from the most ancient times of the human experience that ancestors, departed Masters, and "spirit guides"—of all kinds—were invoked and "presenced" by sound-related ritual, be it drumming and dance or chanting—again, of all kinds. In early cave rituals, generation after generation left their handprints on the cave walls so that, when they had passed, their presence could be summoned back by the community. This explanation, taken from the famous Swami Vivekananda's "Talks on Mantra and Chant," covers it well:

> "The Mantra-Shâstris (upholders of the Mantra theory) believe that some words have been handed down through a succession of teachers and disciples, and the mere utterance of them will lead to some form of realisation. Different Mantras, when they are thus "living," show different signs, but the general sign is that one will be able to repeat it for a long time without feeling any strain and that his mind will very soon be concentrated. From the time of the Vedas, two opinions have been held about Mantras. Yâska and others say that the Vedas have meanings, but the ancient Mantra- Shâstris say that they

have no meaning, and that their use consists only in uttering them .... when they will surely produce effect in the form of various material enjoyments or spiritual knowledge. The latter arises from the utterance of the Upanishads."

Thus, the power of "the secret words" and the power of the ancestors and the ascended Masters "presenced" and absorbed by the practice of mantra.

It is within the profoundly intertwined cosmology of Yoga that we can understand this kind of mysterious "transmission," which so many of us have experienced. Mantra is heard beyond the ears or the body and, somehow, is absorbed by the soul–by the Ten Bodies–beyond space, time, or even cause. Science itself acknowledges in its study of mantra the difficulty of understanding this. Scientific studies identify the "Psycholinguistic Effect (PLE)" by which real physiological changes happen in relationship with sound–and especially not with just *any* sound, but sounds with particular acoustic properties, with complex meanings within their narrative message, or when uttered in rhythmic repetition.

Scientific results on the therapeutic effects of these particularly help us to identify the reality of this "transmission." Examples are French Academy of Science studies of body healing and reducing symptoms of heart disease, Imperial College of London studies of optimizing blood pressure and adrenaline levels, and University of California studies of stress reduction and strengthening of the immune system. Numerous other studies also have involved treatment of addictions. In all these cases, the positive effects appear related to the Psycholinguistic Effect (PLE) noted just above, a matter which has been studied in more detail at the Cleveland Clinic. Most noteworthy regarding the frontiers of PLE are studies with the official support of the European Union in the emerging therapeutic field of "audio-psycho-phonology." This new field directly addresses the still rather mysterious relationship of sound and the body, especially regarding therapeutic attributes across ranges of acoustical properties and the role of rhythmic repetition, as typical of chant.

Across this landscape, be it the useful explanation by Swami Vivekananda, what we know from narratives of the ancients, or the current studies of modern science, we understand the view across all the traditions that mantra and chant "carry power," thus the millennia of "invoking"–bringing in–these participations from such mysteriously shrouded realms across space and time. Thus, in so many traditions, the proliferation of mantra, both personal and collective, comprised of utterances of specific meaning or not, is directly experienced as part of the Divine's spectrum of revealed Wisdom and Truth.

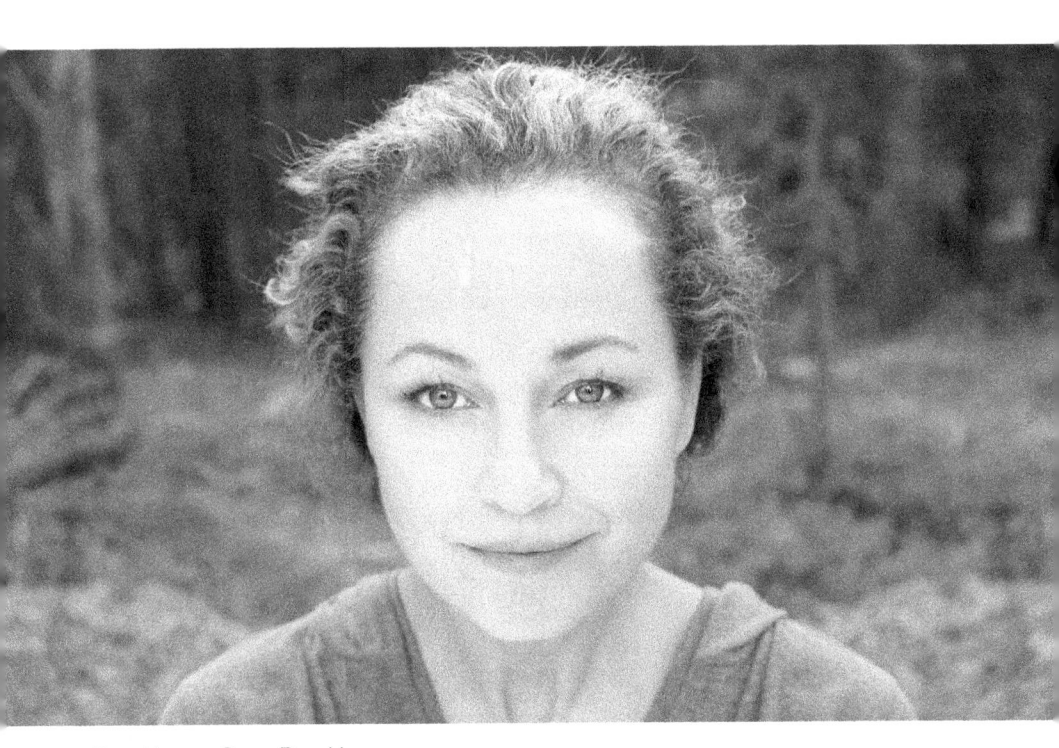

Ong Namo, Guru Dev Namo

Kirtan

Now that we have talked about music and mantra, we can say more about Kirtan. Kirtan creates such a wonderful bridge between the ancient and the now because we live in a time where today's Kirtan musicians are wonderfully well known and even celebrated across our cultures—names like Krishna Das, Bhagavan Das, Wah!, Jai Uttal, Snatam Kaur, Deva Premal & Miten, Jim Gelcer, Jyoshna, Aindra Das, Gina Sala, Guara Vani, Har Anand Kaur, and so many more. You have even seen them on the internationally televised Grammy Awards. Many of them are also my friends, as I have sponsored and hosted their music along with Yoga events, working regularly with Mirabai Ceiba, Mata Mandir Singh (*Japji*; *Sadhana*), Singh Kaur (*Crimson Collection, Vol. 1-5*), Chardi Kala Jatha, and many others. Sat Nam!

Kirtan is rooted deeply within the previous discussion of Yoga, music, and mantra and intricately intertwined within the cosmology of Yoga. The pronunciation of Kirtan comes from the English version of the Sanskrit word *Kirtana*. This is of interest because, as in the discussion of music and mantra, *kirtana* actually means "reciting" or "speaking about" or telling a story. Historically, again as noted in my comments about mantra and music, Kirtan is also used to refer to call and response and also chant. These are all ancient traditions across the Eastern religions. In tracing the history of these traditions, it does not take long to find dance, and then accompaniment of traditional instruments, all added in. What became "Kirtan" thus quickly became a community activity.

Because of its emotionally and spiritually evocative power, Kirtan became especially popular in the Bhatkti period of Yoga's history, growing more and more elaborate with varying mixtures of musical instruments, dance, oration, theatre, audience participation, and, ultimately, a social container for a tradition's collective narrative. As a major community affair, Kirtan requires recognized leadership.

This is the function of the *kirtankara* (or *kirtankar*). This leadership, depending on the size and context of the celebration, coordinates the musical instruments, like harmonium, *veena* or *ektara* (stringed instruments), *tabla* (one-sided drums) and other drums, (*mridangam* or *pakhawaj*), flute and other woodwind instruments, and cymbals (*karatalas* or *talas*).

Kirtan can be performed in all kinds of contexts and settings, and its character will vary with those. In the deepest of sacred uses, it is performed in the sacred houses of worship across the traditions. In the Sikh traditions where Kundalini Yoga is rooted, this means in the Sikh temples (Gurdwaras) where a special feature is the recitation, singing, or even more elaborate performances from Sikh scriptures and historical legacies. One of the most famous Kirtans in history was performed by the famous Bengali Yogi Paramahansa Yogananda who became famous in the West for his book *Autobiography of a Yogi*. In 1923, he led a Kirtan before 3,000 people at New York City's Carnegie Hall. Another setting that so many in the West have become familiar with are the Kirtans performed by members of "Hari Krishna"– the International Society for Krishna Consciousness (ISKCON) founded by Bhaktivedanta Swami Prabhupada and prominent in the 1960s. In that era, ISKCON performed Kirtan in airports, rail stations, and city parks and city centers–also handing out free copies of Swami Prabhupada's *Bhagavad Gita As It Is*. This practice is still a part of many Hari Krishna communities around the world. Philip Goldberg's wonderful book *American Veda: From Emerson and the Beatles to Yoga and Meditation How Indian Spirituality Changed the West*–which I spoke of in my earlier History of Yoga– provides a fascinating account of that era when Yoga was "coming west."

I also told you that my own life's journey into Yoga came first from the music of Kirtan. So, you know how dear to my heart and soul is the music of these traditions, which truly is a portal into the very depths of the mystical and Divine.

Beloveds Among the Global Kirtan Community

As a special addition to this sharing with you, I've created an Appendix—after the Yoga Practice Appendices—that is full of my personal recommendations for mantra, chant, music, and Kirtan. Personally, I've been so privileged and graced by being able to host and co-host programs with many of these great artists. Particularly—in the context of my own personal life and ministry—my experiences have been extraordinary. And I am equally indebted to those who have provided Kirtan directly for the Kundalini Yoga and meditation training programs of which I have been a part.

I also bow to, and unreservedly recommend, along all the others in the Appendices, these greats who are always available to us virtually and, when we have been blessed, in person.

In Appendix 12, I list my favorite recommendations for music to accompany Kundalini Yoga practice, and also my favorite albums for personal enjoyment and spiritual and lifestyle support.

Sadhana

I first noted "Sadhana" in the history of Yogic practices, and then again in my Inspiration and Practice "Becoming Zero Over and Over Again." The first instance pointed to the meaning of the word in its biggest sense—as arguably the most prominent collective and communal practice across the spiritual traditions, especially of the East. In "Becoming Zero Over and Over Again," I concentrated on the individualized setting and context of Sadhana. Sadhana has both these meanings.

I also underscored Sadhana just above, when I introduced the roles of meditation, music, and mantra in Yoga. Each is a part of Sadhana practice both in its collective and individual contexts.

Thus, Sadhana deserves special attention, and for myriad reasons. Let me first reach your soul about it by sharing one of my favorite definitions of Sadhana: "Anything that makes your heart sing."

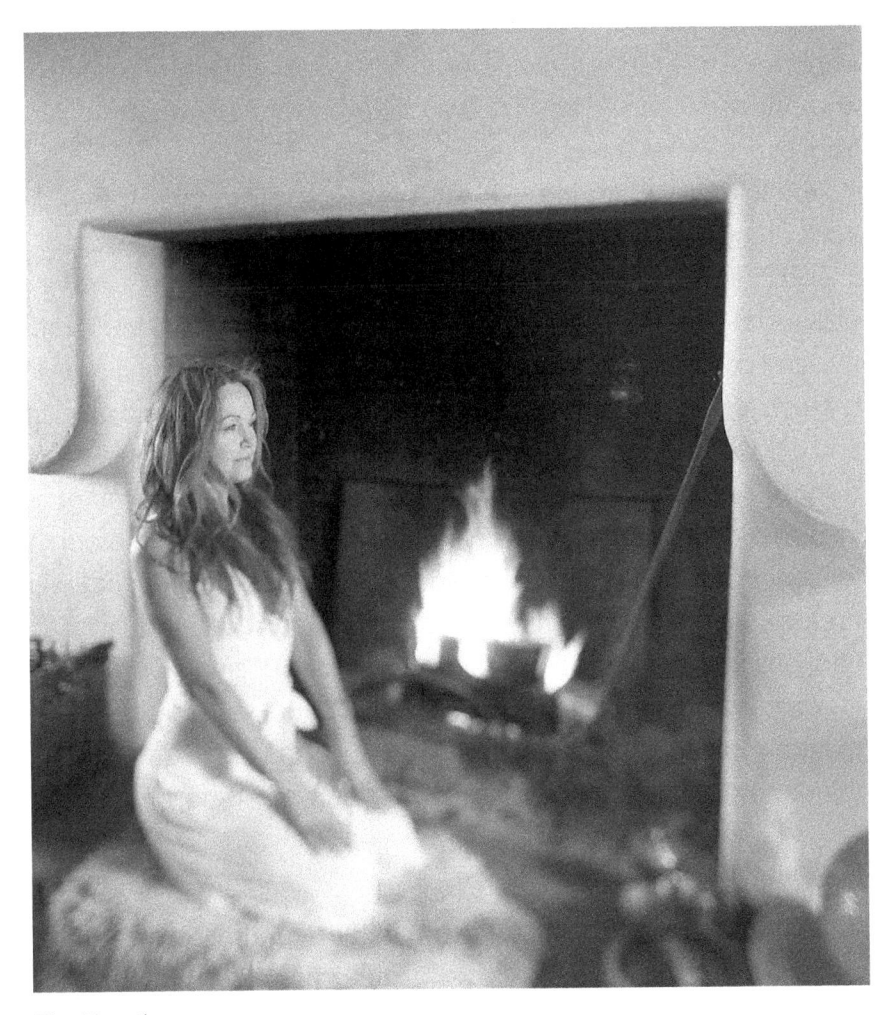

The Hearth

Sadhana's Many Faces

Let's start by looking at the multiple meanings of the word itself. After all, the word—in one language equivalent or another—has been around for at least three thousand years, and across multiple cultures. In all these cultures, the word is both common *and* important and, further, always embraces both its larger (collective and cultural) meaning and its personal importance for the individual Yogi or adept "on the path."

You will find reference to it across the narratives of all the traditions of the Indian subcontinent, and of China and Japan. Secondly, in all these cultures, it always refers to *both* its employment individually, or let's say "in small portions," and its role in the grander collective and communal practices of all these traditions. Perhaps a great metaphor to think of with Sadhana is "food." It can be consumed and enjoyed in small, quite private settings and portions, or in large, sumptuous public banquets characterized by expansive varieties involving many persons and many hours. That's a good metaphor for seeing Sadhana as "food for your soul," energizing your actions, dreams, and goals. Another good metaphor about the faces of Sadhana is to think of it as either singing alone or singing in a choir.

Your individual practice *is* "Sadhana" and so are the larger cultural practices that specifically bear its name. Let's talk about the generality of Sadhana, culturally collective *and* private, first.

Sadhana as Primal Food

I said earlier that Sadhana—in its private or cultural setting—is our opportunity to dive deep and find the central compass points of our souls. It is these compass points that give us both a sense of our soul *and* a knowledge of our own unique path—our sense of what we're called to do. This is why Sadhana practice is so central in Kundalini Yoga.

Collectively, Sadhana is the name for the gathering of the Yoga community for meditation and practice, in the very early morning, actually before dawn. Lasting some two and one-half hours, the practitioner employs that time, in their own private space, or as spaced at intervals across the community's sacred space. Like Kirtan, and Kirtan is usually a part of Sadhana, in community, Sadhana is also guided by the Teacher. This is because Sadhana is actually a very grand sequence of kriyas, and attention is paid to the thematic and inspirational content of each Sadhana gathering. As both an intimate collective and personal practice, Sadhana is a crucial "deep dive" opportunity for every Yoga practitioner. Thus, no wonder the word has definitions in more than a half dozen languages across our Great Wisdom Traditions.

In its simplest meaning—as a noun—Sadhana, it is often simply a synonym of "meditation." As a verb, it means "to form," to "accustom," to "train," or even to "subdue" (from The Hinkhoj Hindi-English Dictionary). In deeper spiritual usages, it means "a means of accomplishing something" and, as such, is attributed to "any spiritual exercise that is aimed at progressing towards the very ultimate expression of one's life in this reality" (that from Wikipedia). Similar, deeply spiritual, definitions call it a *tool*, a tool for our well-being whereby bondage becomes liberation (also from Wikipedia) and, even further, that which elevates to perfection (the Collins Dictionary). Since I've referred over and over in this book to Yoga as a "toolkit," these definitions strike close to my heart.

Sadhana, individually or collectively, creates that environment where you can return to your zero point. Sadhana creates a nest, or landing zone, into which can drop the soul inspirations, discernments, and determinations, allowing you to move forward on your path step by step.

Sadhana as Path and Destination

I think I've said enough about Sadhana that you will always think of it both in the context of individual practice *and* community practice. It is in these combined contexts that Sadhana always serves the same purpose and has the same goal, the pathway to the birthright—Awakened Life.

Of course, this creation of the landing zone, or nest, for your own soul occurs in every action of spiritual practice, but it is especially true of Sadhana practice as it is dedicated *precisely* to that role. It is also a link to community because, when you have found that support within *yourself*, it's likely you will also find it from others, and those "others" who show up in your life will understand and support you.

This is because Sadhana, whether seen in the individual or community perspective, always means *both* the spiritual practice that bears its name and also that its *aim is at a lofty goal*. That lofty goal is Awakening itself.

Accordingly, across the traditions of the Indian subcontinent and on through China and Japan, Sadhana—in one language equivalent or another—is named as the primary practice of these anciently rooted traditions.

In the Vedic traditions of the Indian subcontinent, Sadhana is so synonymous with the path of Awakening that the word is often used in synchrony with Patanjali's Eight Limbs. After all, they lay out the path to, and culminate with, the birthright of Awakening:

> The Eight Limbs of Yoga: *yama* (ethically, what you decide not to do), *niyama* (ethically, the highest choices you decide to make), *asana* (employment of the Yoga postures), *pranayama* (the breathing practices), *pratyahara* (freedom from over attachment to the senses), *dharana* (focus, concentration,

purpose), *dhyana* (meditation), and—the culmination—*samadhi* (absorption, realization, Awakening).

Sadhana is about creating a container into which such inspiration can come. Here, simply, we can just "sit and soak."

When we are in a climate of reverence elements of our True Nature naturally rise to the surface. So, the observance of a time like Sadhana is a "natural" for the receiving of such inspiration and realization—simply leaving our souls open for their birthright and destiny. Here, we can ask those big deep questions that the Great Wisdom Traditions call "self-inquiry":

"Who am I? Who is having this experience? To whom is this experience coming?"

And, received, in your deepest soul, an answer:

"I *am* the universe. This is the universe experiencing itself. I am the universe receiving this—as life and love devoted to *itSelf*."

These revelations were actually those of the great Buddha himself—in the ancient story of him sitting beneath the Bodhi Tree. One version of the story is that, as he was sitting there, he asked himself the question: "When was the last time you were happy?" Then, he remembered an experience he had as a child when he had accompanied his Father into the forest.

Once in the forest, his father told him (in the comforting role as his father/parent, much like "God"), "I have some work to do. Just sit under this tree and enjoy yourself while I go about those chores." As the future Buddha sat there, remembering this earlier permission from his father to "just enjoy it," he had a sudden realization: that everything was fine just as it was, that he did not have to "beat himself up" to acquire spiritual knowledge and enjoy

Being. The future Buddha was quite an ascetic at the time and practicing many severe self-disciplines. As the story goes, when his fellow ascetics later came and found him at the tree, the Buddha said to them of their extreme self-suffering ascetic practices: "You know, we really don't have to do this. Things are fine just as they are, and we can simply enjoy it." Of course, there are many versions of what happened to the Buddha on that day, but this is one of my favorites.

Sadhana in Community

It is no accident that the great traditions have time-tested formulae, formats, and protocols for Sadhana in the setting of community. These reflect ancient wisdom in Sadhana practice following a planned, and generally never changed, sequence. This consistency in community practice is typical across all of the world's great contemplative traditions. This is because, when the structure and schedule of the practice never changes, the attention can be to consciousness itself, and the field of consciousness opened can be extraordinary and expansive. Having the schedule "take care of itself" provides an environment of freedom in which consummate and supreme experiences can "come and land."

This is also true of consistency in spiritual practice itself and especially in your own individual Sadhana. When you consistently take up a daily practice, especially including something as specially choreographed as Sadhana, the very action of being consistent will bring automatic reward. I will say much more about this when I share further about the individual practice of personal Sadhana. But let's begin by explaining community Sadhana, particularly in my tradition of Kundalini Yoga.

As with Sadhana in communities from many Eastern traditions, the formal community Sadhana in the Sikh Kundalini Yoga tradition includes the practice of rising before dawn and, in what is usually a two and one-half hour observance, an empowering sequence of spiritual practices to welcome in the day. Generally, the two and one-half hours derives from it representing one-tenth of one's entire day—as you may have already guessed, reflecting the nearly universal religious concept of "the tithe," the giving of 10% of your life, your wealth.

Kundalini Yoga Community Sadhana

In the formal traditions, like mine in Kundalini Yoga from the Sikh tradition where Sadhana has been cultivated for millennia, the usual morning Sadhana looks something like this. If you take up the practice of Kundalini Yoga community Sadhana, it will vary somewhat depending on the size and context of the community group, ranging from smaller and less elaborate observance (like with *a cappella* chanting or with recorded music to background or accompany movement and mantra) to larger and more elaborate observances (like with live music or even Kirtan).

Special emphasis is put on atmosphere and decor, which can be variously elaborate but, in any event, is always carried out in silence, except for actions performed together. The space in which Sadhana is shared is sacred space, whether it be in the larger, more formal temples (Gurdwaras of the Sikh traditions) or in chosen spaces in homes, communities, retreat centers, and so on. Ample space is left between the participants so that they may have private space for both their silent pondering and also their shared Yoga activities. Traditionally, if from the Sikh tradition, dress is in white, with clean clothes, preferably cotton, and, traditionally, heads are covered. A shawl may also be advisable for warmth and resting (*savasana*). Feet are bare, and usually one sits on a mat, blanket, or other personalized floor covering to insulate from the floor. You can bring a water bottle. Temperature is best moderate, and there is attention to reverent lighting, especially to be in tune with that of time of day. You may want to bring a small flashlight to assist in your reading of the scriptures. The ambience of Sadhana is one of reverence, as, usually, the atmosphere of formal Sadhana reflects that of a holy space, particularly at those celebrated within the formal Gurdwaras.

There is a leader who choreographs and orchestrates the sequence of activities. The leader can be accompanied by musicians or other presenters and, ideally, sits on a slightly risen stage so that the heart level of the leader is at the eye level of the Sadhana participants.

Personal preparation is also important, beginning when you rise in the morning to prepare for Sadhana. This is when you'll want to prepare your clothing and person for Sadhana. Kundalini Yoga adepts in good health traditionally take a cold shower as they prepare to go to Sadhana. This not only is personally invigorating but has been shown by science to increase blood circulation, boost alertness, enliven metabolism, and increase the endorphin chemicals in the brain that are related to peak psychological and spiritual experiences.

The observance begins (often at 4 AM or as publicly announced) with private pondering of the scriptures. It may be quite dark in the room, so, often, such examination of the scriptures is either in dull light or with the assistance of small, personalized lights. In the Sikh tradition, this is the *Japji Sahib*, private readings from the venerated *Guru Granth Sahib*, the sacred scriptures of the Sikh tradition that date to the 16th Century. These sacred texts were added to through early centuries of Sikhism and now comprise some 1,500 pages and nearly 6,000 "verses." Much of these texts also has been, over the centuries, set to music or chant, so the tapestry of recitation, chant, mantra, music, and movement that can be generated around them for Sadhana observance is quite exquisite. Again, as I told you when I shared my personal story, it was precisely this combination of sacred words and music that drew me to what has become my lifetime as a Kundalini Yoga adept and Teacher.

The part of Sadhana reserved for pondering the sacred scriptures reflects wider a tradition across all the world's religions. In Latin, it is known as *Lecto Divino* (the reading of the Divine). There is deep wisdom behind it, as there are aspects to it that benefit the participant devotionally, psychologically, and spiritually. The first benefit is the centering and focusing of the mind on the texts, one of the primary techniques of meditation—concentration. Second is the spiritual benefit of experiencing reverence for the texts, the "looking to something sacred." Third is the understanding, from all the world's traditions, that the scriptures (as with mantra) are "alive," as I quoted Swami Vivekananda, and "carry" the spiritual energy, the "akasha"—history, lineage, and spiritual power—of the tradition. Sadhana is all about this kind of "presencing," like when you feel called to sit quietly in front of a sunset or stars at night, or even before a particular painting in an art museum, and you just "sit and soak."

At around 4:20 AM, the private pondering of the scriptures is followed by the traditional "Tuning In" for Kundalini Yoga practice (as described by me in "The Foundational Elements of Yoga Practice" earlier in this book, and in more detail in Spiritual Practice Appendix 1.

Tuning In is followed by Yoga asanas and/or kriyas for some 20 minutes, generally chosen by the leader of the Sadhana, followed by deep relaxation for five or so minutes, in silence or with quiet music. Lighting is adjusted in synchrony with the advent of daylight, and, at around 5 AM, there is up to an hour of chant, *a cappella* or accompanied by either recorded or live music (depending on the size and context of the gathering) and then meditation.

The observance ends at around 6 AM with a prayer and then the song "Long Time Sun" and what are called "long Sat Nams." These are also detailed in Spiritual Practice Appendix 3. There is then usually a period of "break" followed by community breakfast and fellowship. It is truly an amazing way to start the day and part of the deeply satisfying lifestyle of Kundalini Yoga practitioners around the world. With the sublime fulfilments Kundalini practitioners receive from Sadhana daily, especially the direct experience of Divine transmission, they value the practice with deep reverence.

Personal Daily Sadhana

It's good that you've been introduced to *Sadhana* in general, and in community *Sadhana* in detail already, since, as you can imagine, personal Sahana is really a "mini" version of Sadhana tailored by you exactly for your personal needs and life situation. Of course, you'll want to capture and preserve as many elements from the larger collective Sadhana practice as you can and bring them into your own. Four things are important to remember:

1. *That it be personally meaningful.* You'll want how you chose to do personal Sadhana to be as meaningful and transformative as possible. Remember my earlier favorite definition for Sadhana—whatever makes your heart sing!
2. *You'll likely follow much the same format as community Sadhana—because "it works."* Remember that Sadhana is about building a container into which inspiration can come. There is ancient wisdom in the practice following its planned, and quite never-changing, format. All of the world's great contemplative traditions understand that when the internal schedule of a spiritual practice never changes, even more can come and "land" in your experience—because there is a freedom in having the schedule "take care of itself." This is

also true of consistency of practice. When you consistently take up a daily practice, especially something as specially choreographed as your personal Sadhana, the very action of being consistent will bring automatic reward.
3. *You'll want to create your own devotional space.* You will likely want to create an "altar" or other center of focus where you will regularly practice your Sadhana. This will be an adventure because part of it will involve you discerning what really appeals to you and inspires you for a personal devotional space. Your personal familiarity and attention to this space will be vital to your Sandana experience.
4. *Always do something daily.* Remember to always do something, even if you cannot devote time to a full Sadhana. You will find that this attention to your devotion will evolve and enhance naturally so that you, step by step, discover something that is truly special for you.

The Importance of Personal Sadhana

It's important that you know your own Teacher's commitment to Sadhana. Writers and teachers of Kundalini Yoga note that it is central that Teachers are persons with a dedicated Sadhana practice. This is because only by having cultivated their own personal growth and progression through regular Sadhana practice will Teachers be aware of the subtleties of discovery that naturally arise in this powerful spiritual container. By having traced their own ongoing personal growth and discovery through Sadhana practice, a Teacher can truly be a guide for others exploring and navigating their own unique paths.

Sustaining the Yogic Life

The cosmology of Yoga includes elegant attention to how we sustain the health and well-being of the human body. Here, the traditions of Yoga reflect a larger background of ancient knowledge concerning health, well-being, and wisdom historically known as "Pranic Healing." It includes a variety of health-related modalities anciently rooted in the East—across the Indian subcontinent, China, and Japan. Among these are Ayurveda (and Ayurvedic medicine), the varieties of traditional Chinese and Tibetan medicine, and related techniques like Acupuncture, Reiki, Therapeutic Touch and Massage, Reflexology, Polarity Therapy, Breema, and so on. Today, practices associated with Ayurveda comprise as much as 60-80% of health and medical practices across many nations of the East. They are also practiced in the West, with widely varying degrees of supervision and licensing, along with related practices and derivations of Eastern origin like Acupuncture and Reiki and Shiatsu, which each have their own acupuncture methods.

The practices and knowledge of Ayurveda and Ayurvedic medicine are discussed as early as in the Sutras of Patanjali and within the scriptures (*Vedas*) of ancient India. The roots of these traditions go back much further, however, at least in oral accounts from India dating some 5,000 years ago. Archaeological evidence also has been found suggesting pranic methods as ancient as 10,000 years ago. In Yoga cosmology, *prana* is the general term for understanding the energy-related structures and flows within the body. Today, the global variety of health modalities related to Pranic Healing and, thus, allied with Yoga cosmology, include Ayurveda, Acupuncture, Reiki, Therapeutic Touch, Reflexology, Polarity Therapy, Breema, Qi-Gong, and T'ai Chi. Because of the interest of modern science, psychology, and medicine in meditation and mindfulness, many pranic modalities are now well-studied by neuroscience, showing how closely related they all are, in beneficial effects, to the meditative and contemplative practices of the West, in Judaism, Christianity and Islam. Indeed, such studies show the positive therapeutic effects of pranic methods on respiratory and nervous system function, heart health, and all the documented benefits I described in my earlier chapter "Meditation, Mantra, and Music."

In Yoga cosmology, the connection of pranic practices to Yogic practices comes in the understanding of the Gunas, which I introduced to you in my chapter on Yoga Cosmology. The Gunas are the fundamental states (or qualities) of the senses and of mind, which are in relationship with the five fundamental elements of which all things are made—the Tattvas. These five Tattvas are the ones familiar across most of the world's ancient knowledge—Earth, Air, Fire, Water and Ether. But there is far more to the meaning of these five categories when it comes to their metaphorical meanings and descriptive capacities in our human experience.

- *Earth*, means all things that are Source and at the root or ground being of any thing or activity.
- *Air*, or *Wind*, means anything that is change, development, movement, and energetic activity, dryness, maturity, life supporting. It makes speech possible.
- *Fire*, means anything that animates life, creates or ignites warming and heat, energy or activity, and, in the deepest sense, clarity of consciousness.
- *Water*, means all that flows, penetrates, has continuity which entails flow—timeless, ongoing.
- *Ether* (*Akasha, space*), means all things Formless and yet in creative potential, at once entailing emptiness, communication, formlessness, creative potential, and intelligence.

These, the Tattvas, are what then interact with the world of the senses and lenses of the mind—the Gunas. Considering:

1. the Root Chakra, focused in the rectum,
2. the Generative Chakra, focused in the sexual organs,
3. the Navel Chakra,

4. the Heart Chakra,
5. the Throat Chakra,
6. the Brow Chakra, or Third Eye, of insight, and
7. the Crown Chakra, at the top of the head, also known as the Tenth Gate.

The first five of these Chakras correspond directly with the five elements, Earth, Water, Fire (of digestion), Air, and Akasha (ether, or space). In the practice of Meditation and Yoga, one learns to optimize and balance the flow of energy and function within the Chakras, so that one can achieve one's greatest potential, intelligence, and maximum health as human beings.

This is where Yoga cosmology intimately connects Yoga practice and lifestyle with Ayurvedic health and wellness. Auryveda derives from thousands of years of disciplined attention to patterns, in nature and in humans, and the drawing of conclusions from these patterns, seen to occur again and again. This is what, today, we call "inductive science," and modern science has both inductive and deductive methods. As inductive science, the knowledge of Ayurveda did not originally come from what we call today the scientific method (which method *per se* came centuries later in history). Of this, the *Journal of Auryveda and Integrated Medical Sciences* website (https://jaims.in) notes, "The main difference between inductive and deductive reasoning is that inductive reasoning aims at developing a theory, from patterns, while deductive reasoning aims at testing an existing theory." But, as I've said, in the current global context, Ayurveda is also tested by the deductive scientific method. Ayurveda's patterns, and their repeatability, and thus predictability (both hallmarks of modern science), are likely why so much of Yogic cosmology, and Auryveda, have proven to hold their own with much of today's expanding understandings in science. Thus, globally, culture by culture, we see side by side enfranchisement of these scientific approaches and their applications. The future will be very interesting to watch.

Consistent with the inductive approach of observing patterns and drawing inferences from Yogic cosmology, the ancients of Yogic practice, and the practitioners of Yogic health and wellness today, utilize and draw many of their views from "profiles." The profile approach is also a scientific one. For instance, in criminology, also a process of finding out what is true, profiling is important, and professional profilers make good livings predicting what will turn out to be true from a profile—their view of what patterns mean. That will help you to understand how Yogic health and wellness knowledge draws so many conclusions about the universe, life, health, and human behavior from its profiles of people—what they look like and how they act—matters all profiled in relation to the details of Yoga's views about life, the universe, and you and me. On this background, we can review the basics of the Ayurvedic view, standing on its own history and integrity and using its own terminology.

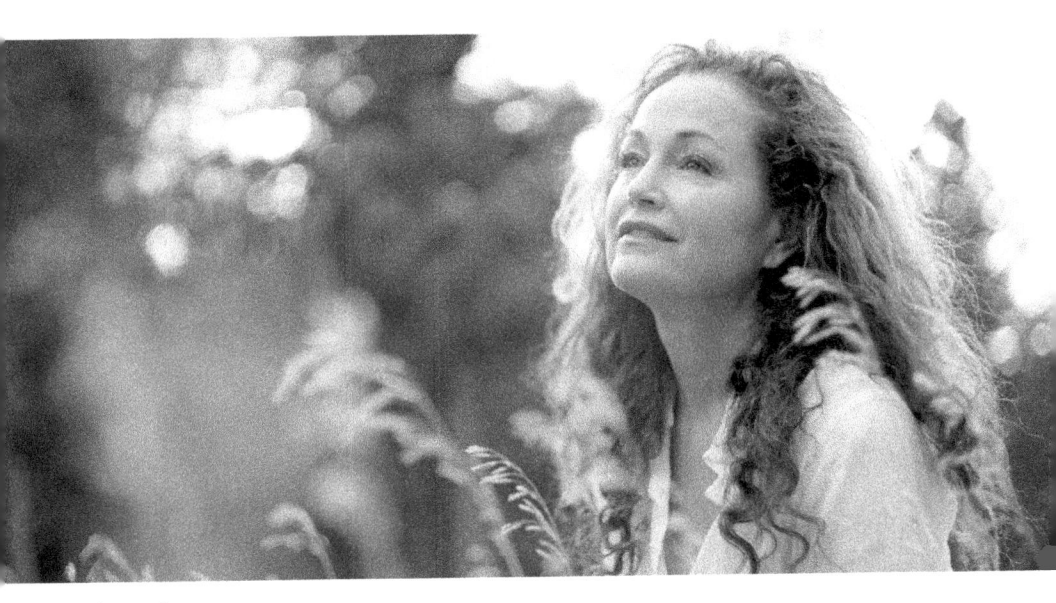

Acceptance

Ayurveda – Yogic Health

Recognition in Yoga cosmology of the Gunas (*sattva*, *rajas*, and *tamas*—the elements of mind and the senses) deeply informs its views of human behavior. Its generalities, or truths, about human health have been learned through centuries of observing humankind and recording the profiles of the general patterns seen over and over again—that is, truths. Thus, profiles—truths—have been chronicled over the centuries with regard to the landscape of the Gunas and Tattvas. If we remember the Gunas from my earlier chapter, we can infer behaviors rooted in each:

- *Tamas*—the basic sense of sensory mind, our raw senses of things (external sounds, and images, but also the internal ones of feelings, even subconscious reactions);
- *Sattva*—the Awakened (Buddhi) mind, which comprehends clearly, discerns well, and sees what is true, even in the largest infinite senses; and
- *Rajas*—as "Ahankar" (the ego sense), in which we experience a sense of identity, sense of self, and "who we are versus others."

Tamasic behaviors are those more primitive—based on need, desire, or instinct. Sattvic behaviors are actions of clarity and mastery, expressed by an interconnected, lively, light, and effective life. Rajasic behaviors are willful, forceful, and directional.

When you then associate these qualities, or lenses of the senses, with the five Tattvas—the fundamental elemental states of matter and mind (and all of their meanings)—you recognize that how these Gunas and Tattvas interplay well-describes the landscape of human behavior and, thus, influence, or even determine, the quality and attributes of anyone's life.

- *Earth*, all things that are Source and at the root or ground of being of any thing or activity
- *Air*, or *Wind*, anything that is change, development, movement, energetic activity, maturation, support of life, breath and language
- *Fire*, anything that animates life, creates or ignites warming and heat, energy or activity, and, in the deepest sense, clarity of consciousness
- *Water*, all that flows, penetrates, has continuity which entails flow—timeless, ongoing
- *Ether* (*Akasha, space*), all things formless and yet in creative potential, at once entailing emptiness, communication, formlessness, creative potential and intelligence

In these interplays, the senses are the filters through which our experiences generate and "happen." When intertwined with the elements and states of matter of which everything is made, our experiences through these lenses determine the characters and condition of our lives. As you will remember from my chapter on Yoga Cosmology, the worldview of Yoga calls this character and condition of our lives—our degrees of clarity or confusion, ease and dis-ease, and happiness or misery—our *samskaras*. Given the ancientness of Yogic philosophy, and the age-old question of humanity and its religions about how and why suffering occurs, we can understand the origin and profundity of this view of life based on the interaction of: (i) the nature of our senses and mind (the Gunas), and (ii) the varieties of "stuff" of which things are made (the Tattvas).

Thus, the foundation of Ayurveda comes from this unified view of the fundamental elements of Yogic cosmology with millennia of observing the dynamics of behavior and health in human beings. The resulting wisdom concerning human health and well-being is the foundation of Ayurvedic practice and all the related Pranic Healing methods of the world. The value of this ancient knowledge is currently enjoying a great revival with the wisdom of these traditional understandings being assimilated into all of our world's cultures. Your reading this book is a part of that.

Personality Types in Ayurveda

Given the interconnection and interplay of the Gunas and Tattvas, Ayurveda's millennia of observing human life graduates from understanding basic modes of behavior to, in sum, describing categories of personalities. In the resulting profiles, tamasic personalities are violent, aggressive, jealous, greedy, thoughtless of others, and generally unconcerned with spiritual pursuits. Rajasic personalities are excitable, preachy, judgmental, and often intrusive into the affairs of others. Sattvic personalities are calm, centered, compassionate, generous, and kind and generally mind their own business. Similarly, Ayurveda also draws generalities about human body types.

Body Types in Ayurveda

The observed body types drawn from observing the interaction of the Gunas and Tattvas are called the *"Doshas."* They include three general, fundamental body-mind types or constitutions, each including a synchrony of physical, emotional, and behavioral attributes.

These three constitutions, or *Doshas*, are called: *Vata*, *Pitta*, or *Kapha*. Let's look at each:

Vata: In vatic constitutions, the physical body is thin with prominent features, tending to be of cooler temperature and with dryer skin. When unwell, the issues are often digestive, with maladies associated with dehydration like constipation or cramping. Persons of vatic constitution are, at best, vivacious, imaginative, and even intuitive. They may favor activities involving movement and fun. At worst, however, they can experience nervousness and anxiety, be emotional and moody, and have a lifestyle that is disordered and with an irregular schedule. If nervous problems persist, they can manifest hyperactivity, sleeplessness, headaches, and lower back pain.

Pitta: In pittic constitutions, the physical body is usually of average build, the skin is fair, and generally moist, and the hair is thin. Lifestyle is usually orderly and structured, including regularized eating and sleeping patterns. At best, pittic personalities are intelligent, articulate, disciplined, motivated toward achievement, and sometimes perfectionists. Emotionally, they can be warm and caring. At worst, they can be intense and quick-tempered, even angry and aggressive. When unwell, they may evidence disruptive conditions like acne, hemorrhoids, heartburn, and gastric issues like ulcers, gastritis, liver issues, and high blood pressure. These conditions, of course, mirror the fire and water tattvas associated with this dosha.

Kapha: In kaphic constitutions, the physical body is of large build with pale, cool, and often oily skin. Hair is thick and often wavy. Emotional tenor is usually slow, relaxed, and easy-going, often associated with eating slowly, sleeping long, and procrastinating. At best, kaphic personalities can be warm, tolerant, affectionate, and patient. At worst, they can become reliant, even possessive, egoic, self-indulgent, and greedy. When unbalanced, this can lead to obesity and fatigue. Maladies may manifest like high cholesterol, sinusitis, bronchitis, and other inflammatory conditions. Such kapha conditions reflect the water and earth association of this dosha.

Of course, because we are made up of what we eat, foods also are recognized in profiles related to the interrelations of the Gunas and Tattvas and the personality and body types.

Ayurveda and Food Types

In Ayurveda, the foods we eat are also classified according to the interrelations of the Gunas and Tattvas. Some quick notes about the Ayurvedic profiles regarding foods readily show their consistency with the cosmology underlying the Ayurvedic views of personality and body types. After my "Reflections on Ayurveda" below, I'll be sharing with you a variety of recommendations from my own experience, just as I did with regard to music and Kirtan.

> *Sattvic* foods reflect the meaning of the word *sattva*, meaning "the mode of goodness." Sattvic foods include fruits, grains, nuts, peas, beans, leafy greens, other vegetables, and yogurt, butter, milk, and fresh cheese. If you are a Yogic vegetarian, these foods should make up the bulk of one's diet, and, in Yogic cosmology, this enhances tendencies toward beneficial spiritual study and understanding. If you are vegan, the view of sattvic foods is somewhat different. Vegetarians don't eat meat from animals, including pigs, chickens, cows, fish, and all others. Vegans, however, in addition to not eating meat from animals, also do not consume other products derived from animals like dairy milk, dairy cheese, or eggs.
>
> *Rajasic* foods reflect the meaning of the word *rajas*, meaning "the mode of passion." Rajasic foods are often more extreme

as to their being more pungent, spicy, sour, salty, or sweet. Yogic diet suggests these foods should only be eaten in moderation, the observation being that they stimulate our egoic tendencies and enhance self-absorption and needs for self-gratification.

Tamasic foods reflect the meaning of *tamas*, which means "the mode of ignorance." Tamasic foods include meat from animals, flesh, alcohol, or any other food whose processing involves death, decay, or putrification. Thus, even sattvic or rajasic foods naturally become tamasic with time. According to Ayurvedic cosmology, tamasic foods make it more difficult to cultivate our spiritual knowledge and lifestyle, since tamasic foods by nature are very demanding on the body. They are more difficult to digest and often lead to systemic maladies in body organs like the liver and digestive tract. Generally, tamasic foods are avoided or used in great moderation by those pursuing a spiritually aware life.

My summaries above about Ayurveda's roots in Yogic cosmology, it's worldview and ancient and modern practices, have aimed to give you a basic understanding of its landscape and how deeply anchored it is in the ancient heritages of Yoga. Deeper pursuit of Ayurvedic knowledge, or its diverse therapeutic modalities, can be a life-long pursuit. Across our world's Eastern cultures, schools, libraries, treatment facilities, and even research institutions are devoted to it, about which I will say more in my Reflections below. In the West, on both sides of the Atlantic Ocean, similar institutions are seeing rapid growth. As you have likely already observed, it is a long-term and global process for worldviews about health and wellness, each originating from far-flung and vastly different cultures, to find their modern integration on the global stage. But this is the process we are in today as our planet seeks to express itself as one, planet-wide, cosmopolitan culture.

Reflections on Ayurveda – with Spiritual Practice

It is sometimes said that Yoga came to the West but Ayurveda stayed in the East. There is some truth to this, but it has also been changing in recent decades, as nearly all western nations have been swept by movements toward more holistic and integrated medical approaches. Some of these directions have resulted because knowledge resources by nature are international today. And not only have movements toward more holistic and integrated approaches increased in recent decades, but so, too, have modern knowledge and appreciation of diet and nutrition, organic foods, vegetarianism, veganism, and so on. You can probably remember when your local supermarkets took their steps toward organic products and vegetarian products.

Ayurvedic practices range from wisdom on diet and nutrition to the practices of ayurvedic medicine. Thus, the widening utility of Ayurvedic methods across the West has increased across all these fronts. Much of Ayurvedic fitness and nutritional wisdom has, especially in recent years, followed Yoga to the West. Ayurvedic medicine has been slower to do so. Of course, there are cultural and political issues here. From the time of the British colonial rule of the Indian subcontinent, there was the collision of western and eastern medical methods. Even today on the Indian subcontinent, there are social and governmental guidelines for how western and eastern medicine is used. The major nations of the Indian subcontinent have institutes for study and practice of Ayurveda, as do the armed forces of those nations. Certainly, one thing that has emerged from those activities is the wide recognition of the value of the ancient practices regarding degenerative diseases, stress-related body and psychological maladies, immune system issues, and rehabilitation, in addition to the nutritional benefits.

In the west in recent decades, the works of Deepak Chopra, M.D. and Andrew Weil, M.D. have received the most media attention in the international discussion of Ayurveda and integrative holistic approaches to health and medicine. Dr. Weil, a graduate of Harvard Medical School, is associated with the University of Arizona and hosts the Arizona Center for Integrative Medicine. He is noted for is pioneering work with the Oxford University Press series (the *Integrative Medicine Library*, 2009-2015) which elaborated ed best-practice methods based on both Western and proaches to health, wellness, and medicine. Like Dr. as published a wide range of popular books, and h I will note in my recommendations below. Most are *Spontaneous Healing* and *Eight Weeks to* n the area of nutrition and fitness, *Eating Well Healthy Kitchen* (with chef Rosie Daley), l and Chopra are perhaps among the ering area of global "cross-over" of , wellness, and medicine, but, in dia Welch, Kimba Arem, and with Dr. Chopra) have also

ental in advancing 's over eighty-five ve dealt with the tivities of the nce firsthand

ard certified in sm and is a Fellow mber of the American

Association of Clinical Endocrinologists, and a clinical professor in the Family Medicine and Public Health Department at the University of California, San Diego. His more than 85 books have been translated into over 43 languages and include numerous *New York Times* bestsellers. His recent books include *Metahuman: Unleashing Your Infinite Potential*; *You Are the Universe*, (co-authored with Menas Kafatos, Ph.D.); *Quantum Healing (Revised and Updated): Exploring the Frontiers of Mind/Body Medicine*; and *The Healing Self* (co-authored with Rudolph Tanzi, Ph.D.).

Dr. Chopra, with colleagues of diverse expertise, have created the Chopra Center for Wellbeing, the Chopra Foundation, and the Chopra Library. They host both www.deepakchopra.com and numerous high-profile international events like the annual "Sag and Scientists" global gatherings. My *Light on Light Magaz* featured Dr. Chopra on the cover of our special issue on *Cha Makers* (www.issuu.com/lightonlight). In these areas, Dr. C has been a planetary trailblazer and, thus, widely recognized the international media as among the ten most influential figures in the world.

My Recommendations

A characteristic of Ayurvedic practice is its bei oriented toward individualized needs. This is why its integrated with Yogic practice. I have already expla commonalities of Yogic and Ayurvedic cosmolo are based on the same worldviews in which harmonizing of mind, body, and spirit. Each su one's physical and mental wellbeing throug like to say that Ayurveda gives us the map subtly, but it also allows us to understand p infinite force to animate and project thro presents a real blueprint for understa organism in an informed, practical, elegant, and poetic way. It is one of the great explorations of Yogic Practice and Lifestyle to investigate and utilize as you continue your journey.

So, as I did with music and mantra, I want to share my own recommendations for your further study and practice.

First of all, for Spiritual Practice. For balancing the elements of the body-spirit recognized by Ayurvedic cosmology, I recommend, and teach, a number of special practices. Three of them I have already featured in this book in my "INSPIRED MESSAGES *with Yoga Practices*" section. So, in your exploration of Yoga and Ayurveda, I invite you to now revisit those sections, and their attendant practices in the "Yoga Practice Appendices," and really take a deep dive into:

- From *Healing Grief*: Balancing the Five Tattvas (the Five Layers Within) – SaTaNaMa [Kirtan Kriya]
- From *Interiors and Exteriors*: Balancing, with Nabhi Kriya with Prana and Apana
- From *Grace and Gracefulness in Transitions*: Nabhi Kriya

These will not only enhance your comprehension of the unified cosmologies of Yoga and Ayurveda, but they will also allow you to experience firsthand the benefit of spiritual practices directly associated with the comprehensive and profound insights of our world's Yoga heritage.

Second, regarding Ayurvedic health, wellness, and nutrition. Let me share my further recommendations about the study and pursuit of the Ayurvedic practices associated with Yoga. I have co-hosted a number of programs with Karta Purkh Singh Khalsa, (Ayurveda) A.D., D.N.-C, R.H. of the International Integrative Educational Institute (IIEI). The IIEI is a school for natural healing which provides herbalist training, nutrition certification programs, and courses for the general public. The IIEI provides training in a diversity of herbal traditions, from Traditional Chinese, to Ayurvedic, to Western herbalism. Dr. K. P. Singh Khalsa is of the foremost natural healing experts in North America, and, at the Institute, you will find a variety of in-person and online courses with offering for beginners to advanced students.

I also want to recommend certain books, and cookbooks, that are now dear to my heart, and I have found to be especially rich and helpful in this life and health exploration: at JoyfulBelly.com, Autumn-Winter Recipes: Joyful Belly School of Ayurvedic Diet & Digestion; *Raw: the Uncook Book: New Vegetarian Food for Life* by Juliano Brotman and Erika Lenkert; *Far Eastern Cookery* by Madhur Jaffrey's; *The Greens Cookbook: Extraordinary Vegetarian Cuisine from the Celebrated Restaurant* by Deborah Madison and Edward Espe Brown; and *The Tasajara Bread Book* by Edward Espe Brown. Also of interest to you will be Banyan Botanicals (banyanbotanicals.com) for Ayurvedic oils and blends based on Ayurveda Diet *dosha* types, and supplements from IHerb (Iherb.com) and Prime My Body (primemybody.com).

Of course, I recommend the books of the prominent Western medical professionals who, as I noted above, have written pioneering work on Ayurveda and integrative and holistic approaches to health, wellness, nutrition, and medicine. Among Dr. Chopra's over eighty-five books, those directly elaborating Ayurveda health, wellness, and nutrition include: The *Power of Awareness*; *The Healing Self* (co-authored with Dr. Rudolf E. Tanzi of Harvard University); *Perfect Health*; *Quantum Healing*; *Return of the Rishi: A Doctor's Story of Spiritual Transformation and Ayurvedic Healing*; *Ageless Body, Timeless Mind*; *Boundless Energy: The Complete Mind-Body Program for Beating Persistent Tiredness*; *The Path to Love: Spiritual Strategies for Healing*; *Reinventing the Body, Resurrecting the Soul*; and *Creating Health*. In addition, Dr.

maladies, immune system issues, and rehabilitation, in addition to the nutritional benefits.

In the west in recent decades, the works of Deepak Chopra, M.D. and Andrew Weil, M.D. have received the most media attention in the international discussion of Ayurveda and integrative holistic approaches to health and medicine. Dr. Weil, a graduate of Harvard Medical School, is associated with the University of Arizona and hosts the Arizona Center for Integrative Medicine. He is noted for his pioneering work with the Oxford University Press series (the *Weil Integrative Medicine Library*, 2009-2015) which elaborated integrated best-practice methods based on both Western and Eastern approaches to health, wellness, and medicine. Like Dr. Chopra, he has published a wide range of popular books, and bestsellers, which I will note in my recommendations below. Most well-known of these are *Spontaneous Healing* and *Eight Weeks to Optimum Health* and, in the area of nutrition and fitness, *Eating Well for Optimum Health*, *The Healthy Kitchen* (with chef Rosie Daley), and *Healthy Aging*. Drs. Weil and Chopra are perhaps among the most well known in this pioneering area of global "cross-over" of our globe's heritages about health, wellness, and medicine, but, in recent years, women writers like Claudia Welch, Kimba Arem, and Sahara Rose Ketabi (who works closely with Dr. Chopra) have also become prominent, among many others.

Undisputedly, Dr. Chopra has been instrumental in advancing the understanding of Ayurveda. Ten of Chopra's over eighty-five books, many of which have been bestsellers, have dealt with the practical utilization of Ayurveda. The worldwide activities of the Chopra Centers have allowed thousands to experience firsthand the benefits of Ayurvedic practices and therapies.

Professionally, Deepak Chopra, M.D., F.A.C.P., is board certified in internal medicine, endocrinology, and metabolism and is a Fellow of the American College of Physicians, a member of the American

Association of Clinical Endocrinologists, and a clinical professor in the Family Medicine and Public Health Department at the University of California, San Diego. His more than 85 books have been translated into over 43 languages and include numerous *New York Times* bestsellers. His recent books include *Metahuman: Unleashing Your Infinite Potential*; *You Are the Universe*, (co-authored with Menas Kafatos, Ph.D.); *Quantum Healing (Revised and Updated): Exploring the Frontiers of Mind/Body Medicine;* and *The Healing Self* (co-authored with Rudolph Tanzi, Ph.D.).

Dr. Chopra, with colleagues of diverse expertise, have created the Chopra Center for Wellbeing, the Chopra Foundation, and the Chopra Library. They host both www.deepakchopra.com and numerous high-profile international events like the annual "Sages and Scientists" global gatherings. My *Light on Light Magazine* featured Dr. Chopra on the cover of our special issue on *Change-Makers* (www.issuu.com/lightonlight). In these areas, Dr. Chopra has been a planetary trailblazer and, thus, widely recognized across the international media as among the ten most influential spiritual figures in the world.

My Recommendations

A characteristic of Ayurvedic practice is its being especially oriented toward individualized needs. This is why its use is so often integrated with Yogic practice. I have already explained in detail the commonalities of Yogic and Ayurvedic cosmology. The practices are based on the same worldviews in which one deals with the harmonizing of mind, body, and spirit. Each supports and nurtures one's physical and mental wellbeing through diet and lifestyle. I like to say that Ayurveda gives us the map not only physically and subtly, but it also allows us to understand precisely how to get the infinite force to animate and project through our being. Ayurveda presents a real blueprint for understanding the whole human

Chopra wrote the Foreword for David Simon, M.D.'s well-known program for optimal wellness: *The Wisdom of Healing, Natural Mind Body Program for Optimal Wellness.*

With regard to diet and nutrition, Dr. Chopra also has published these informative and helpful books: *The Chopra Center Cookbook; The Chopra Center Herbal Handbook: Forty Natural Prescriptions for Perfect Health; What Are You Hungry For?;* and *Perfect Weight.*

All these are in addition to Dr Chopra's noted books on cosmology, like his most recent *MetaHuman* and *You Are the Universe* with Menas C. Kafatos, Ph.D. Drs. Chopra and David Simon also have written a book specifically on the relationship of all this—health, wellness, and cosmology—to Yoga: *The Seven Spiritual Laws of Yoga: A Practical Guide to Healing Body, Mind, and Spirit.*

Dr. Andrew Weil's well-known books which can also be helpful to you include the bestsellers: *Health and Healing; Spontaneous Healing; Natural Health, Natural Medicine; Eight Weeks to Optimum Health; Eating Well for Optimum Health;* and *Why Our Health Matters.* He and Chef Rosie Daley also have provided this book on food and cooking: *The Healthy Kitchen.*

See You in the Kitchen

Along with all the tips above, in Appendix 12, I share with you my own favorite recipe for "Yogi Tea," the essential drink accompanying Kundalini Yoga practice. Adding our attention to food and drink in the context of Yoga cosmology and Ayurveda is another frontier you will undoubtedly savor, and further pursue, as your Yogic life deepens and matures, so I've been happy to share all these tips!

In sum, gauging our progress in this journey we have initiated from the beginning of this book, there is much to be explored as we graduate from our exploration of Yoga into serious practice, an engaged Yogic lifestyle, and the landscape of the ancient knowledges of health, wellness, fitness, and nutrition from Yoga and Ayurveda. As you deepen in your Yogic practice and your understanding of Yogic cosmology and lifestyle, it is natural—likely inevitable—that your interests and directions will likely further move to greater examination and experience of Yogic health and wellness in the foundations and practices of Ayurveda.

COMMUNITY

THE WONDERFUL GIFT OF COMMUNITY

Worldwide today, people are universally saying that "community" is more important to them than ideas and even more important than religious or ideological belief. If you "google "Community is Connectedness," a common moniker these days, you'll find over eight million entries. There are even official definitions (in dictionaries and encyclopedias) for "Community Connectedness" and "Connected Community." Curious about this, I just did a word count in this book so far, and I have used the word "community" 53 times!

To cite some numbers (from the PEW surveys at pewforum.org), some 70% of people worldwide said that "connection" to family, community, and also nature gave them "a great deal of meaning." When asked the same question regarding a religious or ideological belief, the range of that same affirmation was only 20-30%.

It's obvious why. Community is all around us; community *is* connectedness! Just try standing, anywhere, and look around. You are surrounded by a context, a setting, a community. Community is also within us. Turn the spotlight on *yourself*. Our bodies are communities. Your arms and hands carry the food to your table to eat; your legs get you there. Your eyes, nose, and ears assist by their senses, and your brain tracks, maps, and remembers the whole experience.

It's obvious in Yoga. In Yoga, you are utilizing one part of your body in concert with, or support of, of another part. Remember, when I outlined Ayurveda and health, I elaborated on the countless elements that make up and affect our bodies, and this is true not just of our bodies "as is" but also what we put into our bodies every day with what we eat, drink, and breathe. Food and drink also come from communities! When we imbibe food and drink, they flow into communities living inside ourselves. I'm sure you've seen the internet articles and YouTube videos demonstrating how, if we go deep inside ourselves, our body's systems are supported by myriad communities of micro-organisms. These have been living inside of us and have been teaming up with our body's functions for millions of years. Take a microscope to your skin, and you'll see tiny (but cute!) little mites living there, making sure your skin is clean by using any foreign matter as their food! "Creepy," I know, but a further testament that life is community.

On top of this, we are always sharing with each other. There is no way around it. With humans' emotional, psychological, and spiritual dimensions, "community" is lifted to an entirely new level. In fact, what distinguishes humanity from all other creatures on earth actually *emerged* from being in community. Community, and our innate abilities to develop communication, led to speech. Speech led to writing, and, in only about fifty thousand years, human beings became creatures of "culture," a word nearly universally defined as "all the collective manifestations of human intellectual achievement." Look around. No one else builds houses with windows and heating and plumbing! We're quite unique!

Further, if you have never thought of this before, take notice of the walls in human houses and buildings. They are usually appointed with paintings and photographs. Of what? People, communities, and nature. Our deep sense of community was birthed from, and reaches back *to*, the larger breadth of all of nature itself, and, immediately recognizing it as family also, we call it "Mother Earth" and "Mother Gaia." No wonder Indigenous peoples consider all of Creation "our relatives."

Looking Inside Community

So, what are the values of community? Since we are, by nature, creatures of community, let's take a look inside human community and see what makes it tick. First off, scientists studying animals differentiate "community" from "casual companionship" by how much real care a group actually has for its members. Similarly, in humans, psychologists differentiate "community" from "casual friendships" by the same criteria. This question of "how much care" or "how much love" a community has for its members becomes quite unique with humans because humans share stories and, in sharing stories, shared purposes and goals then come into play.

What is also unique about human communities is the variety of ways by which they can initially bond and then further bind together! When human communities have a sense of shared group identity, it serves as a binder. When psychologists assess communities, they actually define these kinds of "binders" that particular communities display. Because of language and stories, communities can also have expressly stated group purposes and goals. With these elements in play, communities can then share in experiencing *achievement* of those purposes and goals. That provides communities with a profound sense of collective fulfillment. These same community "binders"—shared identity and goals—*also* serve to bring in new community members. Accordingly, communities can morph into grander and grander fulfillments of sharing and achievement.

So, with us humans, "birds of the feather" don't just flock together, as the cliché says. They identify and bond because of shared purposes and the mutual achievement of goals and fulfillments.

My friend Charles Vogl won a Nautilus Award for his book *The Art of Community*. In *Light on Light Magazine*, we devoted an entire issue to "Transformative Communities" and portrayed them in light of what Charles had discovered. In the Preface of his book, Charles said that his wisdom and discoveries came from his own years of searching for what real human community was. He was a graduate of Yale Divinity School but chose not to be ordained in a particular tradition where, as he said, boundaries about identity, and the sense of who you were, had already been set up. Rather, he wanted to strike out on his own and discover how authentic communities actually form, and what makes successful ones tick.

Charles noted that statistics show that our current human generations are the most lonely ever. Whereas a few decades ago, nearly two-thirds of Americans usually belonged to clubs of some kind, now nearly two thirds don't. Further, as we know, many of the most current generations have turned to handheld, and other, electronic devices as their method of human "connection." The question is whether real love and caring within a group—the actual definition of community—can be actually satisfied this way. In recent years, this question has become a major social concern.

Turning our attention to Yoga communities, it is my experience that Yoga and community are quite synonymous. They become synonymous because the very practices and goals of Yoga aim at the true measure of community—how much love and care a group has for its members.

This becomes apparent, when we look at Yoga communities through the award-winning criteria in which Charles elaborated about authentic and successful communities—criteria that are *the same* whether a community is a "sacred" or "secular" one. If we match his criteria, see the initial phrases in the bullets below, to what Yoga communities feel they do, see the subsequent phrases in parentheses, the matches are obvious.

- Shared sense of identity (in Yoga communities, "communing together with the Divine")
- Shared values and ethical aspirations (in Yoga communities, "practicing goodness")
- Sense of a higher value to be attained (in Yoga communities, "the path to Awakening")

When we match the kinds of activities Yoga communities carry out with Charles' list from authentic and successful communities below, the matches are even *more* obvious.

- Members join and stay because they feel welcome.
- Members do meaningful things together.
- Members share a meaningful space or place.
- Members embrace shared narratives or stories.
- Members share objects that have deep symbolic meanings.

Here, I ask you to think back to my sections on "Yogic Life." This perspective on community brings even more meaning to these shared activities of Yoga and their lofty attributes.

Furthermore, what is so special about Yogic community is that the purpose and goal of the practice and pursuit itself is aimed so high. Yogic community stands out because of the depth of what is being shared. I think this comes naturally because people who have done significant transformative work on themselves–the "Cleaning Up" we talked about earlier–are then "Showing Up," "Linking Up," and "Lifting Up."

Once you trust community, real community, you'll find it taking you where *you've* really wanted to go and with a lot of wonderful surprises! It makes sense of something I've always said: "Yoga is my tour guide!" Not only will Yoga community be an entry point on many wonderful serendipities, but also synchronicities and synergies! You'll likely also discover that real community often knows what's good for you, even when sometimes you don't know yourself. It's like the multiple "second opinion"—and even sometimes a look in the mirror—about where any of us are at with our "Cleaning Up," "Showing Up," "Linking Up," and "Lifting Up."

If we consider the entire landscape of Yoga—all dimensions of Yogic lifestyle from meditation to asanas and kriyas, to the shared special times (like Sadhana), to what we learn of diet, nutrition, health, and fitness—the Yogic sense of community is truly real, and the sense of love among the community is there even when people are geographically far apart. I often say, "These are the people you could sit around with in your jammies."

In a cosmic sense, it shouldn't surprise us that Yoga creates community around us. "Everything that rises must converge," said the famous Catholic cosmologist, Fr. Teilhard de Chardin, famous for his book *The Phenomenon of Man* and the vision of us "steering toward the 'Omega Point'" (our point of union with the Divine). The novelist Flannery O'Connor made Teilhard's "convergence" phrase further famous with her novelette of the same title. Her book was also a message about the ultimate ends and values of community. In *Everything That Rises Must Converge* (published in 1965, right in the midst of America's civil rights activism), a young white Southerner and his mother treacherously navigate American segregation and, with some courage, learn a deep lesson about human unity and that "the place we meet to seek the highest is Holy Ground."

Community, Service, and Leadership – "Seva"

Later on in this book, I'm going to be asking you about whether becoming a teacher of Yoga, and taking Teacher Training in Kundalini Yoga, may be for you. Since we're sharing about community, I want to share here about the role of the leader, particularly the serving role of the leader, in real community.

"*Seva*" is a Sanskrit word that, in simplest definition, can be taken to mean just "service." But there is far more to it than that, *and,* far more to it than the multiple meanings that Sanskrit words often have. In this case, the very nature of community is reflected in the meaning of the word. The two roots of the word *seva* actually mean "together with," thus, the deeper meaning often ascribed to *seva* is "selfless service." Such service, in its purest spiritual form, involves no desire in the server for any personal benefit or gain in return. For anyone who is intuitive, you will have immediately recognized that *that* kind of authenticity—in real *seva*—could only come from a realization that communities and individuals are actually one shared "Field." In that Field, individuals are only "appearances," albeit Divine ones!

Returning to Nisargadatta Maharaj, the great Vedic teacher, who I quoted earlier in "THIS WAY OUT" of "Going Down the Rabbit Hole":

> "The fundamental fact is that no phenomenal object can have any independent existence of its own... As an actor in this living drama you can only play your role, nothing more. Whatever you may think of yourself, you cannot but be an integral part of the total manifestation and the total functioning ..." – Nisargadatta Maharaj (*I Am That*)

It is no mystery then that one of the most celebrated acts of *seva* in the Sikh tradition of my Kundalini Yoga training is "*langar*"– the serving of food to all, free of charge, without any attention to social or economic status, ethnicity, gender, or religious or political identity. Further, such kitchens are most frequently associated with the temples, or Gurdwaras, thus pointing clearly to the spiritual idea that there is a "sense of a higher value to be attained." I listed this above in our definitions of authentic community.

This is also where true leadership comes in, as it is often with the life of the Yoga Teacher as the selfless server. Often, it is the Yoga Teacher who steps in—much like the mythological Lone Ranger, with his personal face covered—to serve the wider community. And note! He, or she, is immediately recognized in this higher role, and the community knows "help has arrived." In the Lone Ranger myth, he is recognized by his mask, white horse, and even his silver bullets (silver, historically, believed to ward off all evil). Everyone recognizes that cosmic help from the Teacher because the Teacher knows the Sangha is yearning for real community. That yearning is a natural part of the True Self and what the Heart, in everyone, yearns for. As much as happiness is our birthright, supportive and fulfilling community is also our birthright. We are all yearning for communication and community.

Community *is* connection. In community, we have each other, and we hold each other. With the Yoga Teacher, it is not just that he or she strives to know, emulate, and embody the deepest gifts of Yogic practice. The Teacher is also the one who uniquely has an individual relationship with everyone in the community. An authentic Teacher is thus dedicated to the very purpose of real community—that the members of that community experience being valued and loved. Moreover, with Yogic community, it goes even beyond this because the Teacher also wants each community member to realize their birthright to Awakened life and that this is a unique phenomenon in each one. Thus, a true Teacher takes up a unique role in the unfolding of authentic community, with all the attributes we have emphasized above.

TIME AND RELATIONSHIPS – NETWORKS OF LOVE

Sometimes, the best way to talk about community is to share a story that not only conveys its full landscape and meaning but also underscores its manifestations as both magical and unexpected.

I had a chance to visit with an array of friends in Colorado who had known my parents for many years. It was a festive 4th of July gathering, high in the mountains at a historic site with gorgeous summer mountain weather. We were sitting out on a front porch amid decor that looked "mid-1800s," so there was a sense of the "old times," and histories, spreading out in every direction.

Rather spontaneously, everyone started sharing remembrances, and each remembrance sparked another. Curiosity about one question led to another question, and that led to clarifying this memory or that—who someone was, what they used to wear, and even what the funniest (or moving) parts of their personalities were. As soon as someone was remembered, someone else was immediately asked about: "What became of 'so and so'? Do you remember____?" That led to stories about this shared outing or that adventure, with hundreds of details about people, places, and things.

When the whole porch was abuzz with such chatter, someone pointed out that there were three generations of this family present and that, often, the "youngers" had never even met some of the "olders." So, that led to: "Did you know _____? Did you ever meet

_____? He [or she] was such a good person; you would have loved him [or her]." Soon, someone appeared with a photo album asking, "Who was this?" and "What was that?" Then someone was answering, and that led to someone laughing: "Oh my God, I'd forgotten that. That is so funny." One could never plan for an arising like this—a rising and a converging.

The remembrances and love that flowed from all these people were amazing and very moving, and anecdote after anecdote was told in such detail—sometimes from events and happenings thirty to fifty years ago. It was an amazing lesson in how love, in all its little details, is so important to all of us, and how people—as they look to the past and into the future—naturally wish each other the best. It was *humanity* at its best and very moving.

Let's think about the lesson here. I immediately think of the word "Reciprocity"—a word, and way of life, that we know is sacred among native peoples. "Reciprocity" is often defined as the practice of exchanging things with others for mutual benefit, or mutual dependence, action, or influence. It is actually innate in our nature. Scientists point out that language itself fundamentally distinguishes humans as creatures of reciprocity. Our human penchant for story-telling shows how wonderfully synergistic this has become.

When you go and talk to loved ones—about loved ones—your own personal stories ignite their personal stories, and a state and feeling of reciprocity and community arises. It also brings out extra generosity in us. For example, I've noticed I find myself often saying to a masseuse after I have received the massage, "Wow, you look great!" when I'm the one that just got the massage! This kind of reciprocity is a very natural and spontaneous projection. It is also very healing. It is a healing event because of the synergy of love arising. So, not only is everything arising and converging, but we are reflecting each other much like mirrors.

We Mirror Each Other

Science today knows about "mirror neurons." These are neurons in our brain that fire when we are doing something with others, especially when participating in similar activities, in partnership, or in synchrony. These neurons are different than the neurons that engage when you are just doing something alone. Further, mirror neurons create a feeling of connection and empathy. Although a lot of this research is new, it helps to explain things like why we identify with sports figures playing a sport, singers singing, dancers dancing, romantic moments in the movies, and so on. We feel a sense of fulfillment in ourselves even though it is not us that is doing the actual actions. Similarly, we also react to the pain and suffering in others as well.

The message here for Yoga communities, and why Yoga becomes so attractive, is that it offers a new experience, one that can be shared with others. One of the ways that we seek fulfillment is projecting ourselves into future situations. Remember the last time you planned a vacation? That is what you did; I'll bet you projected that future event through a number of options and then decided what was best. As humans, we imagine ourselves in a situation. So, we may look at a Yogi, or a community of people obviously happy in their Yogic practice, and we automatically think: "That could be me!" or "Whatever that person has, I want that!"

So, when we start a new program or a new class, or sign up for Yoga Teacher Training, we already have an idea about it—a vision. We are inspired. We want to try something new. Similarly, later, as we have eased into the program, we find ourselves wanting to set goals and achieve them. Once again, scientists say this is another unique trait of humans. Other animals do difficult things because they have to. Humans seem to want to, and they often call this "fun." Remember President John F. Kennedy in his inaugural address in 1961 talking about going to the moon? He said, "We do not do these things because they are easy. We do them because they are hard." This says something important about the intersection of our human and divine nature.

So, this natural reciprocity runs deep. We see grace-in-action in communities who gather around the true aspects of love. In such communities, people are truly respectful of the breadth of real love that is being shared and expressed. This is especially admirable when the object of the love is someone you actually don't personally know. I see this all the time—people reaching out to others in that true spirit of *seva*, selfless love. Love is just love and has a life of its own. As the greatest Seers have said, "Love is communion of Divine Self to Divine Self; it is life and love in devotion to *Itself*." So, people, often strangers to each other, leave such gatherings with a glow, softer hearts, or even milky eyes.

I think of this a lot when a sangha assembles for a retreat, especially if it is one for which they all have traveled a long distance from diverse places and, as yet, don't necessarily know each other personally. It is an expression of great trust in the process of such gatherings that are based on love. They trust each other to all show up, and they all trust the Teacher. This reciprocity then extends to everyone having the opportunity and ability to ask very honest questions and to inquire about what is really on their hearts. What is amazing about this phenomenon is that it is actually happening, and it is a healing process simply by everyone just being themselves.

AUTHENTIC RELATIONSHIPS

We often aren't aware of the many kinds of relationships going on simultaneously in our lives, *nor* their important potential. Let me give two simple examples so you'll recognize immediately what I mean. How many people realize that children actually have three relationships with their parents? Each child has a relationship with their "mother," their "father," *and* their "parents." Each is unique. How many partnered couples realize that they aren't just called to be boyfriend/girlfriend or husband/wife but, when pertinent and needed, also have important roles for each other as brother/sister, parent/child, friend, and creative colleague? None of these important and necessary vertical roles (as parent/child for each other) or horizontal roles (the others above) disappear simply because of age or coupling up. Understanding the kinds of relationships that are going on simultaneously in our lives, and that they have certain features, is important for us in navigating life. As a very wise teacher of mine once said, and it also refers to community: "It's important to know whose problems are whose!"

It's really only within the context of our world's great Wisdom Traditions and perennial philosophies that we get clarity on this. Let's look at "Love" for instance. There are actually many kinds.

Reference books say, depending on how you look at it, there are over thirty kinds of love! But the ancients—from most of our religious understandings, and even those of modern psychology—

settled on six. These are now pretty standard in our social and legal understandings of love. We all experience these kinds of love and recognize their distinctions. We may simply have not thought about them for a while. They are very important in our understanding of the various roles that love plays in authentic relationships.

First, let's look at *"Eros"* or what so many call "erotic love." The reason I discuss it first is that it may surprise you to know that it is not just the romantic or physically passionate kind of love we most often associate with the word. It includes that, of course, but is also about love *itself*, and about beauty. Meanings of *Eros* elevate to include the most beautiful aspects of being including art, philosophy, and, you guessed it, spirituality and spiritual truth. What we experience with romantic love and beauty are actually pointers toward the highest of spiritual truths. That is why so many wise Teachers say that the closest thing to actual Awakening is falling in love. The problem is that we don't know how to handle that experience. We tend to think that love has possession attached to it. So, sometimes Divinity's gift to us—of something very much like Awakening—gets mishandled. We forget, as St. Paul said in the Bible:

> "Love is patient, love is kind. It does not envy, it does not boast, it is not proud. It does not dishonor others, it is not self-seeking, it is not easily angered, it keeps no record of wrongs. Love does not delight in evil but rejoices with the truth. It always protects, always trusts, always hopes, always perseveres" (1st Corinthians 13:4-8).

And *that* gift of love can turn to suffering. Actually *Dukkha*, which we talked about as "suffering" earlier in my chapter on "Healing Grief," also has a much more refined meaning which we can understand so well here. *Dukkha*, the first of the four Noble Truths, actually doesn't mean suffering itself but our tendency, from our ignorance, to make things into suffering. So, yes, it's a Divine gift that falling in love mimics or parallels Awakening, but so often, the experience gets turned into suffering.

Let's look next at the love of parents and children. The ancients called it *Storge* (pronounced *Store-gay* in Greek). It's super-relevant here because you have probably already thought of the parallel of the parent/child relationship and our relationship to the Divine. What characterizes this kind of love is strong and protective empathy, and the loyalty of the parent (or Deity) for nurturing the highest and best good for the child. This helps us to understand that the parental relationship goes far beyond just parent and children. It should be a nurturing love that we can offer to anyone regardless of their age or our other relationships with them. This also is the kind of love and care I talked about in "The Wonderful Gift of Community"–the love a spiritual Teacher has for those whom he or she is leading. Another especially poignant example is when, in the context of long medical term care, and especially hospice, children often "change roles" with their parents and truly become the parent for their own parents, supporting them through their death transition. People report this as one of the most moving experiences of their entire life, and completely unexpected. As you may have already intuited as well, we can have parental love for ourselves, treating ourselves with kindness, patience, and nurturing. In fact, in our busy world today, a modern practice in some Buddhist communities–*Tonglen* or Compassion Practice–invites an individual to "become his/her own best friend" and promise to treat himself or herself with every accommodation and concern of being a "best friend."

Another kind of love agreed upon by the ancients is *Philia* (pronounced Fillia by the Greeks). It is also super-relevant here because it denotes our love of friends or "the love between equals."

This is, again, such an important dimension, no matter what other kinds of love relationships we have with someone. Loyalty, trust, understanding, and creative synergy are also what characterize the best of love between friends and equals.

Let's speak now about the love of ourselves, our love of ourselves as Source's children. The ancients called it *Philautia* (pronounced Filosh-shia in Greek). This love is certainly what the parent wants for the child, or Source for us. It is the love connected to self-esteem, self-confidence, and the courage of believing in ourselves—as I said in the earlier chapter "Radically Being Yourself." On the downside, so often it is *us* that stands in our own way. On the upside, we actually have a dynamic capacity for active love for ourselves. It is not the love of narcissism or ego, but the love of patience and nurturing for us to each reach our highest and best. Many of the most happy and successful people report that, at some point in their life, they promised themselves: "I am going to be my own best friend. I'm always going to assume the best of myself, cut myself slack when I actually need it, and move ahead toward my goals and fulfillment with both patience and confidence." When you have *you* on your side, in the best and purest way, that is an unbeatable combination.

There is another kind of love the ancients spoke of that is so important to our understanding of sacred community—*Agape*. It is the love and concern for someone irrespective of who they are or what their "station" is. It is the kind of love we're familiar with from the story of the Good Samaritan who stopped to help an injured traveler whom he did not even know. It is also the basis of the *seva* tradition of *Langar* I told you about when the Sikh community provides free food to all as a part of the ministry of their temples.

Christianity in particular has made *Agape* (Ah-gop-aa) a famous word. *Agape* is an overarching understanding of love that touches on all the others I have described above. It takes on this all-embracing role simply because it is *that*: all embracing–the big hug I talked about in my first sentence of this book, that "hug" for the relationship of Source and humankind and for brother and sisterhood. It has all of the attributes ascribed to love as noted in the words of St. Paul just above.

It is all these varieties of love that make up the horizontal and vertical dimensions of love that we experience across our comprehensions of this vast universe, and it's important, as I said, that we understand that we are meant to "surf" with them all. They are all at play all the time.

Kundalini Yoga and Authentic Relationships

The Kundalini Yoga tradition has a unique and rich background of practices that reflect the balance and expression of love across the human community. Specific practices embrace the individual, the coupling of the masculine and feminine, and the understanding of shared energies across and among the community. These make the practice of Kundalini Yoga in groups, especially with the support of music and mantra, uniquely inviting and deeply moving. There is a particularly wonderful synchrony in our "knowing" of these experiences from both the heart of the Great Wisdom Traditions and from modern science. There are many aspects to this interplay, and some may surprise you.

For instance, singing is a form of brain synchrony. It uses both sides of the brain together (the left side for lyrics and senses of meaning, and the right side for melody and deep emotion). When such synchrony is experienced by us it releases chemicals in our brains that produce pleasure. Similar synchronies, and related pleasure, also happen when humans move together, as in group Yoga or dance–or even with "a wave" at a sports event. Music and recitation together enhance this effect through a process science calls "vocal attraction" which, science says, is the way birds and other animals "talk" to each other. Such synchronicity goes even deeper, however. In groups, it produces the feeling of identification and happiness within a group, something called "psychological convergence." And, get this, it's even stronger in spiritual groups that are sharing a high ideal and aspirations toward the Divine. These groups trigger what is called "halo effect," something that causes spiritual groups that are truly "walking their talk" to have an "attractive glow" about them.

Obviously, what science knows today was known by the ancients—and it has cultivated the best of our most effective millennial spiritual practices. Kundalini Yoga, for instance, will introduce you to Kriyas that build on the synchronous energy of the community, including practices with partners and pairings of the masculine and feminine. Practices with partners, called "Venus Kriyas," work with the energies of the partnership, producing tangible experiences of co-working and mutual fulfillment. They are further enhanced when a masculine/feminine polarity is involved. After all, this is the structure of the universe!

There are also more elaborate, community-wide practices that involve understanding the synergizing of energy of the whole community. *Sadhana*, which I have already talked about in much detail, is one of these. In *Sadhana*, as I said, a number of things are going on simultaneously, enhancing the journey and maturation of the individual as well as the community. Another important one, about which I will give some fuller perspective below, is "White Tantric Practice." It also directly relates to cultivating authentic relationships by synergizing the energies of individuals *and* the community toward mutual enhancement and fulfillment and, ultimately, the Awakening of all.

White Tantric Practice

I'm sure you've heard the word "*Tantra*" before since you'll find 138 million entries about it at Google!

Briefly, if you generally think of Tantra as "energy," "White Tantra" cultivates and nurtures the subtle realm energies of community members as brothers and sisters, colleagues, and friends. It is "Red Tantra" that has to do with subtle realm energies related to sexuality, and "Black Tantra" where subtle realm energy is used for secretive action, manipulation, or control (even evilly) as in black magic. But the meaning of *Tantra* is not that simple—an important point to make right away.

This brief explanation helps us to further understand how *Tantra* relates to Yogic energies *and* to community *and* authentic relationships. The word *Tantra* in Sanskrit literally means to "compose," "conduct," "connect," or "weave"—or even to "expand" or "extend." Such definitions are a good understanding not only of energy in a community but also of the role music plays! Further, with regard to community and relationships, the meaning of *Tantra* also parallels the meanings for the Sanskrit word *Sutra*. In its simplest meaning, *Sutra* refers to religious texts or writings, as in the famed Yoga Sutras of Patanjali I have spoken of already. But literally, *Sutra* also means "sewing," "threading," or "connecting," again clearly pointing to *Sutra*'s function to unite and serve and bind together the community. Patanjali, in his famous Yoga Sutras said, similarly, that *Tantra* means the tying together of many elements into a whole. So, in the sense of community, and relationships, it all makes sense.

These observations clearly point to how Yoga practice works and serves in community, and particularly as to the highest and best of authentic relationships. So, it is no wonder we frequently hear comments like these about the experience and importance of partnered and shared community practices: "I felt the community supporting me. It is the community, and my partner, that energized me, that pulled me through. It was amazing; without my partner I could never have done it." For these people, the experience has been "real" in "real time."

To understand the depth of the ancient traditions that underpin these effective practices, we need only look at the scriptures of Sikhism from which Kundalini Yoga arises (the *Guru Granth Sahib*):

> "The God-conscious person delights in doing good to others (p. 273); the God-conscious person acts in the common good (p. 273); contemplate and reflect upon knowledge, and you will become a benefactor to others" (p. 356).

SEEING IN OTHERS WHAT OTHERS CAN'T SEE IN THEMSELVES

Every one of us has a potential for change. When we are sitting in Yoga class, we are already sitting in a manner inviting collective transformation. In Kundalini Yoga, the Teacher sits on a stage so that the teacher can see the student but, more importantly, so that the students are at the heart level of the Teacher. This is so essential in feeling each other and being able to respond to what students need and are asking. This further reflects the realities of the shared energies among the individuals and the community. It truly is one Field. Because of this, students commonly come up to their Teacher after a practice and say: "You gave me exactly what I needed today. How did you know?"

Everyone in community is both healing and growing, and it has also been the same for me. Having been my own experiment[!], I've come this route myself. I not only understand but hopefully also am able to share, usefully, everything I have learned along the way. So, whether it be my lessons from growing up; navigating my vocational track (and having been both neglected *and* celebrated and well-known); my experience of the spousal and family track; building a house; my own path with Kundalini Yoga, mystical spirituality and exploration of esoteric traditions and their healing gifts, or even doing some novel things (like my being a helicopter pilot), there is a lot to share. And multi-tasking? We can certainly talk about that, too, since I have multi-tasked through a passionate career as an entrepreneur.

Sometimes, I feel like an old "tinkerer" who has learned by taking things apart and putting them back together. Sometimes, that is how we learn. Each of us is called, through our own experiences, to learn the things we need to–to be able to serve others. Sometimes, it only makes sense when we look back in hindsight. I sometimes imagine this path, so common to all of us, as like riding on the caboose of a train, a train that is pulling us along with our destiny. Sometimes, we are standing on the back railing of that caboose, and the path of the track, from which we've come such a long way, is shrouded in fog, and we can't see it at all. Then, as I'm sure you have experienced too, that fog suddenly clears, and you see, very precisely, how you've come and from where you've come, and it all makes sense.

What's important is to have the courage to stand in "who you are," even when you don't know all the details. It is a spiritual principle that when you are moving from one level to another–and the old stories no longer satisfy, but the news ones have not shown up–that standing firm in "who you are" makes you ready

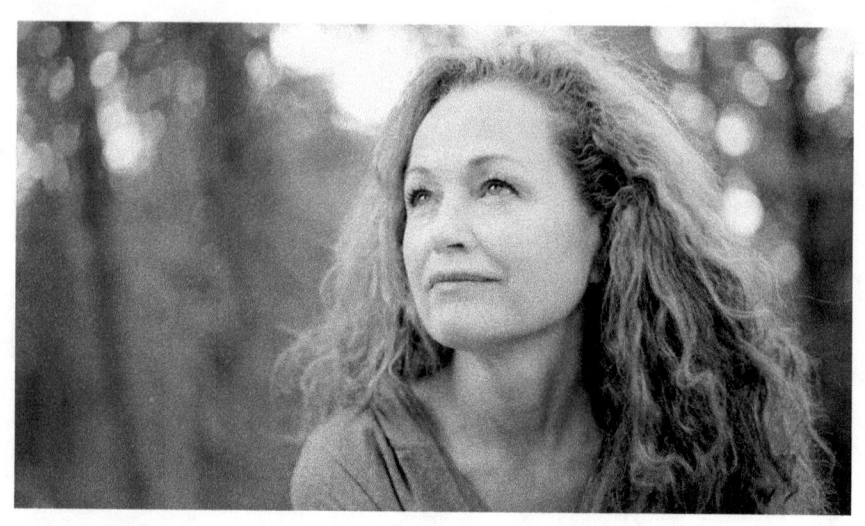

Ask Yourself

for what is coming next from the Divine. Further, when you land in that new place, you also have to be ready again to freely surf, as free as you have been at any level you have already mastered. So, on this subject of "Seeing in Others What Others Can't See in Themselves," you also need to be able see it in *Yourself* and strike out in the direction of that destiny.

Stages of Life

The Ancients had a lot to say about the life stages we go through. They have had thousands of years to observe. Some things are true no matter at what time or in what culture they occur. But things also have changed. For one thing, we live much longer today, giving us chances for more chapters. This is worth looking at because what we're talking about in this chapter is seeing potential—in others and in ourselves—and living accordingly.

To the ancients, there were only four life stages. In the Vedas, they are called The Four *Ashramas*, and they form an interesting and instructive translation for modern life. They are: Brahmacharya (student), Grihastha (householder), Vanaprastha (forest walker/forest dweller), and Sannyasa (renunciate). If we wanted to modernize those four life stages, we might say they are "growing up," "householder," "contemplative," and "reaching Awakening." But I think we'll see below that modern life—also leading to Awakening—has a few more stages, a few more chapters.

"Growing up" is the first stage—childhood and schooling—a long enough story in itself, for all of us. It is always a combination of "stars in our eyes" but also learning as we go. We all know it's a wild ride when it is happening; yet, when we look back, just like riding on the back of that train when the fog clears, it often all makes sense. After "Growing up," it is then the time (to use the colloquial term) to "make it," to answer the question, "What do you want to be when you grow up?" Today, I think we can call this stage "career" (which

I'll use rather synonymously with "making it"). This is when we strike out, with some sense of who we are, to create and build what we feel we've been called to do. This is truly an important and central part of our lives. Here, the roller coaster can really set in–the right decisions and the wrong breaks, or even the wrong decisions and the right breaks. We can invest in things with our entire self, and then lose it all, or we can be carried by some mysterious muse that seems to work for us no matter what we do. Both can happen.

I remember when I was marooned in Paris as not just an aspiring model but one who had been sent there with a contract! Then, it all fell apart. Although I will tell you much more about this in the next chapter, I cried at first but then picked up some fashion magazines and set my sights *exactly* on the photographer/director I aspired to work with–where I felt my hunger for succeeding had met its match. This was, perhaps, my first real experience of digging into *my* vision of "making it"–of my career–and, I think, the first time I had felt that spiritually famous moment of "knowing and not knowing at the same time." I am so grateful now that I was able to make that empowering step. I approached his office forcefully and got an appointment with his agent. Soon, I was the favorite model of one of France's most famous fashion photographers. Today, my photos with him are still in museums and on fashion retrospective websites around the world. *Light on Light Magazine* did a full retrospective on all these museums and fashion websites in 2018. Go to issuu.com, click on the first issue of *Light on Light Magazine* (the early one with me on the cover, arms raised), and head for pages 46-51. I'll tell you more about it when we speak of "Finding Your Way."

Today, it's more often after "making it" that we often move on to be the "householder" that the ancients spoke of. Often, this is when we've waited long enough "to get our act together," and we decide to "settle down and have a family." Note that this pattern is so common today that there are already these popular phrases that characterize it. Sometimes, this is upon us before we're ready. Every story is different, but as I told you in "Letting Go of the Past and Reinventing Your Self," "making it" and householding ran quite together for me. For me, these included the two decades of bringing up *my* family who are all now safe, successful, and happy. Luckily, with our longer lifespans these days, we get some additional chances in life that the ancients didn't really have a chance to see.

The ancients jump from "householder" to *vanaprastha*—the contemplative life as a senior citizen. Back in those days, it was your last chance to use your time on earth to claim your birthright of Awakening. Well, luckily today, we have more time than that. For me, and I think for many others, by the time you're done "making it" and then householding, or the two side by side, you actually have gained a tremendous amount of real maturity.

In this day and age, this opens up a new chapter in so many of our lives where we can really think about serving. In modern life, we have lots of ways we can get from householder to *vanaprastha* (senior), to *sannyasi* (seeker of Awakening), and then to actual *moksha* (Awakened life). This is a time of life in modern times when many people dedicate themselves to their communities, write books, work with not-for-profit service initiatives, and even run for political office. For me, this is when I seriously set out on the path of Kundalini Yoga and became a Kundalini Yoga Teacher.

For many, this is the time to participate in reconciliation. After having jumped through all the hoops of "growing up," "making it," and "householding," it's a time to contribute to larger platforms and larger landscapes of public service. By this time, many of us also have children, or even grandchildren, and they are a wonderful mirror for us to understand the wonder that has surrounded our own path. We can be thankful for all the blessings, look back on the "bad times" with a grain of salt, and just go on with Being and *seva*.

TURNING THE SPOTLIGHT ON YOURSELF

Above, we've moved from community to authentic relationships, to seeing in others what they may not see in themselves, and, finally, to the creative stages of life. We want to move now to "Finding Your Way – By Yourself and with Real Friends." To do this, we first need to shine the spotlight on ourselves. I've wondered when the best time was to share more intimately about my story, the "me" that brought me here. If community is, as Ken Wilber says, "me + you + us + all of us," I'll need to cast my own anchor here before going ahead.

So, where to begin? I knew back when I was 8 years old that I was different than many others around me. Looking back, I was more sensitive than my family could handle. At school, I was always a victim of bullying, not a bully, and I got bullied by both boys and girls. It's hard to know what they might have thought later when my careers blossomed in quite public ways.

So, I cried a lot during my upbringing—I think mostly because all the choices that were made were out of my control. This probably explains why I jumped at the chance to make a major one for myself. So, when I was "discovered" for my future major modeling career, I jumped right in. With a contract in hand, I accepted a one-way ticket to Paris. I just had to answer the call, and I went.

It's quite an amazing story after that, how "fate," "Source," or whatever one might have called it, finally got me to the right people.

Looking back on it, perhaps it was my first lesson in "trusting Spirit." However, as I told you before, the initial contacts who brought me to Paris were a bust. I was picked up by this French guy who thought he could take advantage of me, but something within, call it intuition, told me, "Do not leave the car." Initially, I was dropped off to wait at a pensione, without my luggage and no money. You can imagine what went through my head. "Where am I?" I wondered, and "What have I gotten myself into?"

I ended up sitting at that pensione, missing my family and home. I never was able to obtain my luggage. I had decided to keep a healthy distance from my original "handlers." So, I started living place to place, but still meeting the modeling appointments that were made for me. In Paris, upon awakening one morning on the Rue de Odeon in Paris in the pensione, the feeling of extreme sadness looming had become so apparent I had to make an adjustment after three months of living this rejection. Something had to change. But no one wanted me. What to do? Broken out with pimples, I cried between each audition until one day, laying in the single, tiny share-space of my pensione room, I had an epiphany. It was, as I said earlier, my first experience of digging into my primal sense of what it meant for me to "make it." *I was smart enough to start from exactly where I was.* With a rush of decisiveness, I began paging through modeling magazines until I saw a model, and a design layout, that "looked like me." Looking back from a spiritual perspective, it's like a lot of us when we pick up our first dharma book and begin to find both "our Dharma" and "our Tribe"–our starting point. I said to myself, "This photographer would love me."

As it happens, I'm invited to lunch that very same day, and my girlfriend, another model, sees her agent in the back of the restaurant *Joe Allen's*. I am introduced, and say to this agent, "You look just like my grandmother!" The agent thought that I was referring to her age. However, my grandmother is the most beautiful Slovakian grandmother in the whole wide world! She looks at my friend and says, "Your friend Carrie needs to go immediately to the studio of Guy Bourdin, where he is casting French *Vogue* today." Off I went, lunch forgotten, in my only attire—CU sweatshirt, *Levi's* 501s, and *Candies* famous wooden shoes. Pimples and all, I arrive only to find the most gorgeous, blond, Swedish models in the waiting room for the same audition. GULP! Lo and behold, the Creative Director from French *Vogue*, Patrick, walks towards me (I was convinced he was going to ask me to leave the room) and reaches out his arm and grabs my hand. He then sweeps me away into the imposing presence of Guy Bourdin—where I hand over my portfolio with all of Pamela Hanson's profile photos of me in wheat fields in Boulder. Monsieur Bourdin starts to move through the pages while starring at me only and not looking down at the pictures even once. Maybe he did, but I didn't notice. I just smiled ear to ear for that moment was so surreal in so many ways. He offers me back my portfolio with an *"Au revoir. Merci."* Off I sprint. The next thing I knew, after returning from the audition, I was booked for six months of French *Vogue*. It goes to show you how destiny is at your fingertips when you are willing to answer the call, even if it's not laid out, mapped, or planned. I was kept very busy, so busy, in fact, that I soon had the nickname "Ms. Bourdin!"

As it turns out, this guy was, and is, famous—actually a legend. Today, you can look him up in Wikipedia, and you'll find:

"Guy Bourdin (2 December 1928 - 29 March 1991), was a French artist and fashion photographer known for his provocative images. From 1955, Bourdin worked mostly with *Vogue* as well as other publications including *Harper's Bazaar*. He shot ad campaigns for Chanel, Charles Jourdan, Pentax and Bloomingdale's. His work is collected by important institutions including Tate in London, MoMA, San Francisco Museum of Modern Art and Getty Museum – (https://en.wikipedia.org/wiki/Guy_Bourdin)."

Soon, a well-rounded portfolio of my photos, an assortment of Guy's French collection adorning the pages of French, Italian, and English *Vogue*, found their way to Eileen Ford in New York City, and she invited me back to the U.S.A. to be with Ford Models. Here, I met a supportive professional family and made many close friends. Of course, all of them recommended me to whomever *they* were shooting with, and "Voila!" Soon, I was working all over the place.

But this success brought new challenges to finding *my* way–my making it–in my own unique way. My life became a whirlwind of events to run to and keep up with. How to keep going? In a life that was work, work, work–glamorous as it might seem–there was, personally, nothing to fall back on. Although people in this business meant well, because they were also super busy, they honestly don't have time to mentor or counsel. I had to realize that I had landed in the "fast lane," and it was truly a shock. But this was also the beginning of my learning that we are born of heart and soul and, even deeper than that, spiritual Source–as one dictionary defines it: "the essential quality and character of the cosmos itself, and one's own nature." So, without knowing it, I was being set up to find a spiritual path.

Truth be told, modeling consists of being treasured while your picture is needed and then being left out in the cold. It turns out to be a rather remarkable metaphor for how life runs on this planet without any deeper Spiritual understanding. The job is all about goals and deadlines and the wishes of the people at the top. So, just like in the military, the "grunts" (be they models or soldiers) are brought in very young. "What about me?" doesn't exist. But you do learn to be tough. And again, if you have a heart at all, you realize that all of these people are dear, and sacred, in their own way. So, I did also find many good friends and good people, and my heart never forgets; that is just who I am.

So, this was, actually, the beginning of the life lessons that would lead me to Yoga, spiritual practice, and a journey to spiritual transformation.

A year or so later, I returned to Paris for a job and was standing in front of the Metro doors, which opened in a whoosh. And who should be standing alone there in front of me, as if I had called his soul's essence to meet me, but Guy Bourdin. He paused in the opening, in as much shock as me, eyes meeting one another for the final time on this plane. I smiled wide, as I always had, and we had our last aha! moment, a giggle, as I said, "Bonjour," "Au Revoir," and "Merci, Monsieur!" as the doors shut on the platform. Guy will always remain a true witness to my spirit.

How that Journey Began

Settled in New York City, my apartment was in the West Village on Horatio Street. This was one block from The Integral Center, a center that offered Yoga, natural and healthy foods, and much more. I was settled now professionally, but I had also recognized the rather bleak landscapes of that business as well. I realized I needed to be interested in finding peace and happiness—whatever "those things" were! Looking back now, I can fondly remember the words of the Vedic seer who I have quoted already so many times in this book—Nisargadatta: "You tend to wake up when you've gotten tired of everything else."

By that time in my life, I was smart enough to know that I was entrenched in patterns, sometimes destructive ones, just like the business I was in. As we all know now, life sets up the circumstances for us to move ahead, to take it upon ourselves to find the way through. That in itself is a miracle! So, although I didn't know it at first, the intersection of my life with Yoga was not only the way I could learn to make healthy change for myself, but also for others.

The Dalai Lama is famous for advising that, when challenged, the path to take is often the one nearest our home. So, that is certainly how I discovered Yoga. Also, interestingly, as I began my explorations into self and Source, through my first physical and spiritual "deep dive" into Yoga, frontiers that I could meet and embrace with others also appeared. Without my knowing it, I was being thrust into the world of *seva*—serving for the good of the whole—and an inevitable role as a change-maker.

There were a lot of issues in the modeling business. Jerry Hall and I, and a few others, decided to ask for a meeting with Eileen Ford. We wanted to ask for privacy for the lingerie shoots we were doing, to have the studio to ourselves with no one except the photographers allowed onto the sets. Sure, we were relatively clothed, but it was still "violating" to have all kinds of people there watching. We succeeded in these meetings and established the "closed studio," and we also got an increase in our hourly rate.

Another "movement" I soon found myself pushing was the one for insurance. I was actually in the midst of this advocacy when I suddenly became the guinea pig for it. I broke both of my arms braking and flying over the handlebars of my bicycle to save somebody else who had walked out in front of me on New York City's 5th Avenue as I was heading to a *Mademoiselle* shoot (P.S. Nobody told me that nobody rides a bike in New York City!) I had no idea what had happened, so I lifted up my bike, threw it over my shoulder, and huffed up four flights of stairs where they greeted me and asked why I was laughing. Crying, I responded, "I think I have a broken arm!" They sent me to the hospital, and I didn't even tell the doctor about the right arm until I tried to push up from the table after they cast the left arm, and the right one collapsed! I left in two casts.

I was scheduled to do the Ralph Lauren Fashion Show the next day and had to cancel, but I went to the show anyway, in both my casts, and ended up with more jobs than I had prior to this booking. People felt so sorry for me and hired me on the spot! Regardless of the positive outcome which taught me that you can turn anything into a miracle, it highlighted the issue, and soon, insurance became a reality. The items above are standards today, but they were not when I was first in the business. I'm happy that I pushed to initiate those changes.

Speaking above of *Mademoiselle*, it is important to note that Arthur Elgort, American fashion photographer for the magazine, launched my career from an introduction from Esme, who was one of his favorite models and was considered by me to be the Audrey Hepburn of our time. I remember sitting there with my avant-garde GB portfolio, which looked nothing like the All-American girl for whom *Mademoiselle* was looking, and Arthur said, "Don't worry. We got this." I had many joyful years working with *Mademoiselle*, traveling the world.

I also will always have a soft spot in my heart for Patti Hansen, as she gave me my very first opportunity to work with Polly Mellen at *Vogue* for the designer Laura Biagiotti.

I was soon to learn another lesson of the spiritual path—sudden change. Unexpectedly, I fell in love, married, and moved to London. Out of the blue would unfold a next stage of my life and my own journey in spiritual transformation—*my* life as a householder.

But as I said when writing about life stages earlier, this time in life compressed my householder life and my "making it" life (Part 2!) very close together. As could have only happened by this move to London, I received the placement, for Actors Study, at the Bristol Old Vic Theatre School that I wrote about in "Letting Go of the Past and Reinventing Your Self." I had always been interested in acting, but this was the most unlikely thing to happen. Usually, it takes four years of auditions, but somehow, I got in on my first. This changed my life. They did not care how I looked; they only cared how I spoke!

As this was all unfolding, I was first, a mother of one, and then, a mother of two! So, I was studying Shakespeare, in acting school, and also tending to a family. Sometimes, I was up at 4:30 AM making the family dinners for the day. It was another whirlwind.

I remember the last day of school. My husband, armed with dozens of garbage bags, picked me up. He quickly put all my belongings into the bags and whisked us away in our tiny Mini Cooper. He was obviously glad to have this period of life "over with." I was very appreciative that he gave me this time to find my voice and my destiny. The family that I married into also was at the front of giving women a voice. They gave women a chance to be feminine, built factories that closed doors early on a Friday afternoon so that families could be together for the weekends. Laura, my mother-in-law, was the pioneer to design the first tea towel, to dress women in frocks of soft cottons and other organic fibers after the 60s full of miniskirts and the Biba era, so we could feel cozy and a part of nature comfortably (https://www.ashleyfamilyfoundation.org.uk/our-history). I recognize my blessing every day.

Yoga Takes Deeper Hold of My Life

Eventually, I was back in London. When I came back this time, I decided to start sharing the gift of Yoga with the acting world. In this sharing, I could not only go on with my own healing and transformation but also could share that journey with so many others, especially others who were living lives that demanded the best of them both spiritually and physically. I began teaching Yoga, for actors and especially members of the Bristol Old Vic Theatre community. This, with dear friends, became The Life Centre of

London. If you search for it today on Google, you'll find it says: "The Life Centre: Yoga London–London's original trusted source for Yoga and well being."

My dear friends who joined in starting the London Life Centre gave me an interesting assignment–to meet all the greatest Yoga teachers and invite them to join us for programs at the Centre. So now, I was in the company of bright souls, saints, and loving people who shared new ways of living and was a woman and a mother who was raising my children vegan, homeopathically, and holistically.

Although I was living a pretty devoted and disciplined Yogic life, I originally never thought about becoming a full-time teacher. But then, one day, I met *my* Teacher. Confirmation came through a dream that she was the Mentor for me–"the One." Everything she told me to do, I did, without hesitation. I trusted her, followed her to India seven times, and studied the Art of "Letting Go & Letting God!"

Through Kundalini Yoga and the Sikhs, I learned how to be humble and how to forgive myself, first and foremost, so I would not blame, criticize, or judge. I had to look into the mirror, as if a widow, and see the real me. My damaged ego was put to the ground to taste the dirt in a sweat lodge, and I was to be given the Native American Lakota Name *"Chanté Eton Wo Wa Gla Ka Win"* (woman that speaks with her heart), and then "Karuna" (Compassion). And I have to live up to these names; I did not ask for them.

Even my Sikh name–Livpreet Kaur–required the same dedication, meaning "One pointed to God." I took the leap. I did twelve Level One teacher trainings and raised my kids as a single mother. I stayed in my log cabin house on 150 acres in the forest, and I bowed down to the Mother day after day to give me the courage and strength to beat the odds that were placed against me. I had to get rid of fear because I was brought up with fear.

In every relationship, I took fear with me. How could I trust when no one had taught me? It is a predicament so many of us have found ourselves in, and this is why our pursuit of the spiritual path together is so important.

There *are* Gods and Goddesses and Wisdom and Grace, Energy and Light! These Teachers are Real, and we can find them, and share them. We owe this pursuit to our own Nature, our own Birthright.

Every day, I climb the mountain to my home on a switchback road some 3,500 feet above a valley floor. Nature always welcomes me, whether it is in snow in winter or the sweet warmth of summer, reminding me that I am not alone. There, I find my home awaiting me, my nourishment nurturing me, and my humble heart grateful for all the awakenings of the day.

Every day, I teach Yoga to share a Heart of relaxation, restoration, and trust. Every day, I ask God to give me more patience and forgiveness and less judgment. Every day, I get to meet new souls who are longing to find their original voices again. I can always assure them that, in this long journey, we can find these things because I know it is true.

Miracles are not hiding, waiting for us to find them; they are actually already here, finding *us*. It is a matter of recognition. To find our natural breath, to let go of competing ways and instead to serve with love and grace, creates the same space for all—allowing that same natural process to unfold in all beings. There is room for everyone. Invite that multiplicity into your heart, and let it glow, just like the universe glows with the light of all those stars.

Encourage all, especially younger folk, to be a part of this emerging Global Recognition of Oneness. For the younger ones, we might help make it easier. Yoga is unity, but unity is not uniformity! Perhaps they don't need to learn the hard way, as so many of us did.

Become a mentor, a light worker, a healer. We all have it in us to do so. This is in the Word of God from all traditions: you were born perfect; stay out of your own way and let His/Her hand guide you.

After three decades of Yoga practice, three careers and Motherhood, and my roles now in magazines, books, and audio and visual media, this is what I bring to the story of my life stages, and what it has meant to find and pursue my path. So, this is who I bring to community and the companionship of paths which we'll share more about below.

FINDING YOUR WAY – BY YOURSELF AND WITH REAL FRIENDS

The very thing that binds you to a community or to a relationship–and therefore is fulfilling to your sense of identity and recognition, and your feeling of being safe–can become, if one is not careful, the very thing by which you lose your autonomy, discernment, and freedom and ability to walk into your own destiny step by step.

So, as with so many things, there are two sides to this coin. How are you healthy with yourself, and how are you healthy in community? How have you walked your path when you've had support, and how have you walked your path when that support was not available?

There are so many subtleties to all this, since we can become unrealistically reliable on others, where their healthy dose of support can become unhealthy if we become dependent on it, and vice versa. This co-dependence is the "common cold" of all kinds of relationships–with friends, families, mentors, and careers. It's like how we have to know to take just the right amount of vitamins each day, and not the whole bottle, just because "they are good for us."

We can be blinded by so many things–love, being in love, careers, familyhood, or running around. We've all known people–good people–who are just "lost." They don't have any frame of reference or reference points allowing them to move along, assuredly, step by step. And, of course, cultural norms are also a problem. Cultural norms can create all kinds of challenges when they are out of step with who we feel we truly are. So, it is a maturity when any of us—within ourselves, friend to friend, spouse to spouse, family member to family member—can really ask and answer important questions, and see things moving in that consistency, honesty, and stability I've spoken of herein so many times. This is how one can walk with one's destiny, step by step, and with the full range of support and love from others that is a part of it.

Finding Your Own Voice

Voice is the most valued part of Yoga—how you communicate and how you are received and heard—as a student, as a teacher, as a Divine human being. When your voice has not been heard, how does one open this channel? Yes, chanting for sure. Yet, a deeper exploration has to be heard from within—a longing to be heard. It is one of our most common complaints, and a true one: "I am misunderstood. I did not mean to say that!" or "That is not what I mean. Let me explain." This comes from difficult years of childhood upbringing—being laughed at by siblings, classmates, or even parents; being put in the room and required to shut up or keep quiet (better seen and not heard); living through parents divorcing, etc. These are experiences many of us have had.

In that "Growing Up" I described in "Stages of Life," you discover you can be fine with not explaining yourself so much. People either hear you, or they don't; they "get you," or they don't. There is a sense of relief in that when your voice has been in pain and cannot express itself. Maybe this is why I chose to be a model (or it chose me actually). I could just smile. But I had to learn that that wasn't enough either, because I was still in pain inside while smiling—hurting, missing my dad. That sort of conversation was ongoing and persists in many of us. We are really good actors until we have to audition for something real. Then, the truth wants to start coming out, and we have to cover it up with protection. So, often we "don't get the part," not only professionally but also in our own lives. It hurts to stage your truth.

As I said in "Letting Go of the Past and Reinventing Your Self," it was in acting school where I first began to learn about my own voice because they didn't care about what I looked like. That was a traumatic journey. I remember the first time I went to acting class at the Warren Robertson School of Acting in New York City. They had me play Cleopatra, and "My, Oh my!" I could not even say a word. I was so afraid and embarrassed that I sat in the corner and cried. At the time, I didn't realize that I was afraid to "tell my truth," to open up, and to break through to my voice. Luckily, like with my helicopter pilot-instructor, again, someone believed in me. It takes a very loving, special teacher like Warren or Larry Moss, and my acting coach in London, to see your potential and to give you the encouragement to break through. Sometimes it's tough love, though, almost like an order. The day before my audition at the Bristol Old Vic, my London acting coach said: "You show me you can actually do this!" When my helicopter pilot-instructor simply jumped out of the helicopter and, without warning, left me on my own, he yelled through the sounds of the rotors: "Go solo *now*!" Yikes, there is so much packed inside us! You all know what I mean because you also have been there.

There is a celebrated invocation, unique to the Sikh tradition—"*Akal*" (pronounced "ah *call*")—which addresses this need we have to release, to fly free, and to find our truth. Literally, the word means "timeless," "immortal," and "unlimited." It is used as an invocation and chant at the time of death where it invokes eternity, being, and divine essence. Traditional to all the great historical Gurus of the Sikh heritage, it has a poignant meaning in that tradition, which is the root tradition of Kundalini Yoga. Looking back now on those times when I had to learn to break free, to abandon the old, and to bring in the new, I find myself remembering *Akal*. In the mystical, remember earlier in "Mantra and Music," Vivekananda's explanation of how mantra and "word" are "alive" and "carry something." The great mystics say: *Akal* frees our earthy pain; *Akal* drops the infinite ocean into your consciousness; and *Akal* takes you home. *Akal* is heart and devotion, undying and everlasting. The spirit of *Akal* is what I speak of above, what it takes to trust your own callings and goals and to free yourself to make them a reality. When I think of *Akal*, it spontaneously tells me of its own meaning: "*Akal* is your infinite ocean. *Akal Akal*, my heart is devotion undying, *Akal Akal*. Rain is falling; the Ethers are calling; this soul is longing to fly away; this soul is longing to fly away. Love does not die; it becomes the sky; it drenches the earth, death and rebirth. *Akal*, with your name on my lips, I breathe in this life; with your name on my lips, I reach for the sky. My love showers down eternal, *Akal Akal*." Guru Nanak (1469-1539), the founder of Sikhism, says: "Life is our precious breath, I inhale this gift, I exhale this death, I exhale this death." Kabir, the great 15th Century Indian poet writes: "death doesn't have to repeat, I come back again Mother Earth beneath my feet, mother earth beneath my feet. It's time to go home." Of course, by "death" (Nanak) and by "going home" (Kabir), they do not mean just physical dying. They are speaking of the death of the old insecure and afraid self, and the going home to our true voice, our true path to all we can be.

Experience and choice brought these lessons to me, as I hope it does for everyone else. To the extent I'm not sure that everyone finds the answers they deserve, that's why I'm sharing my experiences here. I have been able to luckily listen to my soul's compass and follow her direction with no bargaining for character benefits. When I struck out on my own, the biggest gamble of my life, and didn't have the usual support to which I had become accustomed, I had my helicopter pilot's belief in my abilities. I was able to become sure enough of myself that I could go into a career where I could pretend to be someone else. And I was able to make difficult decisions about the integrity of my life and who I am, in light of loved ones around me, and survive on my own two feet from the depth of my Self. We all live from assumptions, our sense of what is true. Sometimes, these senses will be wonderfully in sync with others, and other times, we will butt heads.

So, a healthy way to live is to be able to find your way, both by yourself and with real friends. You know the saying: "We live in two worlds—our own, and the one others drag us into." So, it matters how we identify our real friends—with the criteria of honest support, deep trusting love, and the ability for that support and love to adapt with the changes that come inevitably with life. That's real friendship, within ourselves and with others.

Yogic lifestyle creates a foundation for this kind of living by its ability to give life a context by which you can see, and measure, real change—and see and measure your growing maturity. This self-knowledge is an amazing by-product of day-to-day practice. You are no longer just caught in the "tizzy" like a ping-pong ball. Instead, you can have solid anchors, solid measuring points, *and* good people, with the same intents, who will join you there.

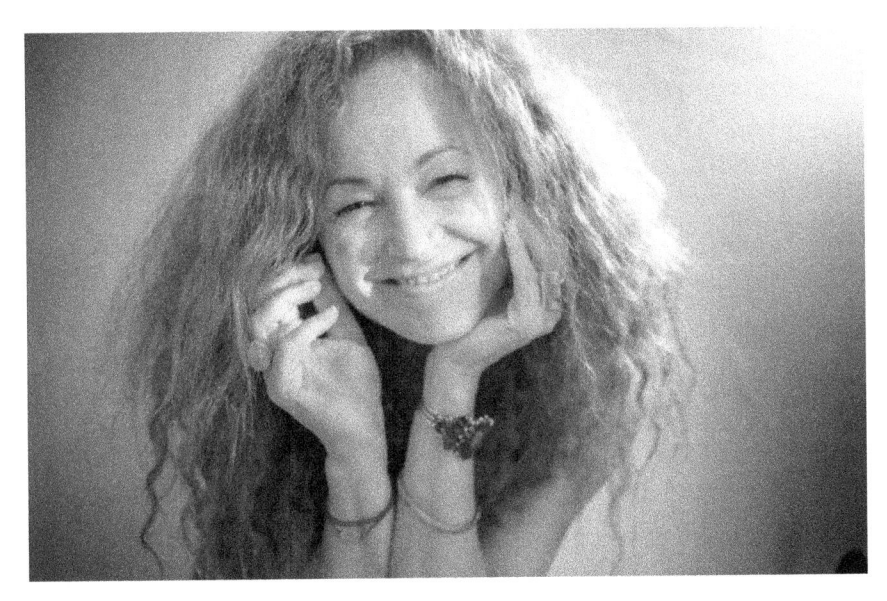

Essence

LOVE IS THE COMMON DENOMINATOR

If you scan the Table of Contents of this book, you'll see the journey we have taken together so far. Just above, we shared some final insights about what it means to arrive at our own maturity and to be confident of, and thankful for, the birthright of an Awakened consciousness. The truth—that is, "what does not change" (the definition I shared earlier), be it mysterious or sometimes not—is that the journey and the journeyer will always be unique.

If we look again at the subject matter that we have explored on this journey thus far and ask what it all has in common, we arrive at the equally mysterious essence that ties it all together—love.

In writing that sentence, I got curious to see how dictionaries define love. The definitions are big and broad, so when you paste several together, it is something like:

> "an intense feeling of deep affection encompassing a range of strong and positive emotional and mental states—from the most sublime virtue or good habit to the deepest personal affection or simplest pleasure"

It's almost as if love is like the blood running through our bodies, that it is really the currency on which our whole life depends.

In one sense, we can look very simply at love—that it basically is the "something" we are all looking for. Something that we all have in common is love. Who doesn't want love? Who would tell you they don't want love? I've never met anyone, or any conscious thing, who didn't want to be loved. Asking who or what might not want to be loved is a laughable question—to all of us.

If we center on this central truth of love, it also truly buffers all the wider concerns we may have like how we assess, or have assessed, how our own life has unfolded. It's natural for us to ask about our lives: "Was it fair? Did I get a fair deal? If there is a God, or Source, was I treated right?" However, from the perspective of love, and from the growing maturity we have talked about throughout this book, factoring in love can change that outlook significantly. From the perspective of love, obstacles and challenges are to be expected and navigated with courage, skill, and grace, not by protest or with poisonous resentment or self-pity. From the viewpoint of love, we understand we're going to be challenged when we start to vision our life and play it out.

From overarching love, we can see the twists and turns of our journey, unique to each of us like the grids and tracks of a gameboard, where each step links to the next and there is unlimited potentiality. We can see the story of our life, especially from the lens of maturity, as a ladder, each rung taking us higher and higher. Often, what comes with that is something unexpected. That "unexpected," as I said in "Becoming Zero Over and Over Again," can be a simple grace, challenge, or twist, or it can be major bottleneck, trauma, unexpected accident, disappointment, or even a broken heart. But it is something that causes our lives "at that stage of the game" to turn around or take a new direction. Like I've said before, this reality is so common to all of us that there is even that phrase "at this stage of the game." We remember the famous boxer saying, "Everyone has a plan until the first punch!" or the sayings, "Life is what happens while you're busy making other plans!" and "Did you ever notice that when the Universe wants to do something it's not too concerned about what else is on your plate?" As a scientist friend of mine reminds me, although nature and life (especially in the movies or in great books) can, in fact, be very beautiful, we also know that nature and life don't just automatically "make everything nice." We are going to have challenges, even very serious ones.

But in hindsight, and from maturity, like so many stories in this book, we can deeply see it all as a serendipity, just like my story earlier about the young man who found his Awakening in a prison, or the metaphor I shared about riding the caboose of the train that is pulling your destiny along and suddenly seeing very clearly, when the fog lifts for a moment, the path down which you've come.

If we go directly to the "I"—the "I am," the "I am *that* I am"—and understand our True Nature as a part of Divinity, we can see that the unfolding destiny of anyone's journey toward their birthright is their own hero's journey. And, as scholars of the hero's journey tell us, it is a journey from "muddle" to "resolution." Every story I have shared in this book has been about moving from "muddle" to "resolution," and, as I've said, we often do that in stages—very natural stages. That is what is so brilliant about Yogic practice and Yogic life. The practice, and the life, clearly delineate the path and the goal and set you on your way, step by step, while also providing the insight and benchmarks to gauge your progress as you go, frontier after frontier, fulfillment after fulfillment, and achievement after achievement.

So, from this biggest picture, we can truly say that the common denominator of it all is love.

The other thing I have said throughout this book is that we each need to take the utmost care of ourselves along this journey—learn nurturing, healthy self-love. The first thing we did together in this book was to remind you of our birthright to Awakened life—and then we shared chapters about "how to" access and attain that birthright. They all boil down to caring for yourself as the sacred vehicle for your journey, even taking up your own body as the tool—the practice of Yoga—and understanding the amazing integration of this body-soul vehicle in the grand context of how the universe is structured and what it's made of. Thus, I shared the gifts of the cosmology of Yoga and its direct connection to the Great Wisdom Traditions of health, wellness, diet, and nutrition. There is no doubt that, in our modern day, Yoga has become a global phenomenon, and there will undoubtedly be further advancement and development of these treasured understandings, originally from the East, as our world now builds a shared, cosmopolitan, global worldview for its future.

As we have said, "connection is community," and "community is connection." Finally, there is not only the dimension of devotion to ourselves as we make our birthright journey toward Awakened life, but there is also constant natural attention to community, that community of mirrors that I talked about in "Time and Relationships – Networks of Love." As we agreed, none of us is alone. We are part of a Field, a field of interconnectedness and overall Oneness. As the poet says, "The river flows through many places—as if to stand still in one."

Certainly, the knowledge of Awakened life, what modern science calls "nondual consciousness"—knowing we are not separate—is what we are made of. We are all made of the same thing, are all part of the same thing, and are all part of the same process. When we know this, we know that *this knowledge*, and then *seva*—selfless service—is all there is.

So, there is nothing abstract or theoretical about love for the individual and love for community. It's "nuts and bolts" or "bottom line." We're talking just about love and nurturing environments of love.

BIGGER LOVE – MOTHER EARTH, MOTHER GAIA

Having declared above that love is the common denominator and that our life is, and should be, about fostering communities of love, we celebrate how deeply Yoga comprehends the sacred vehicles of our bodies, minds, and souls—our part of the Great Adventure of the Cosmos.

In this celebration, let's acknowledge our earlier comprehensions of beauty and Oneness, our first breath at birth and the innocence of our childhoods when we saw so clearly the beauty of everything around us: the winged ones, the four-legged, the creepy crawlers, our fellow humans—wherever we saw, and embraced, that beauty. Often when I talk to the deepest of Gurus and practitioners and they speak of their practice, nearly *all* confide the centrality of their relationship with nature, of their "time alone in nature."

The relationship of nature and spirit, of nature and inspiration, of nature and awe, has been alive across all the pages of this book. It has grounded our discussion and elaboration of the human body, all the natural intersections of our lives with food and drink and breath and the vast comprehension of Yogic cosmology.

As you know, among my many names (each from chapters of my life—Caroline, Carrie, Caroline, Livpreet Kaur, Karuna, Rev. Karuna), there is also *"Chanté Eton Wo Wa Gla Ka Win,"* my Native American Lakota name which means "woman that speaks with her heart." I am an adopted pipe carrier in this Sioux Nation tradition where I am also ordained as a "Wisdom Keeper." I am blessed to live on 150 acres in the high country of the Rocky Mountains. As you undoubtedly know, too, like so many other places in the United States, and around the world, it is an area perennially threatened by the devastation of forest fires. Such fires are part of a larger global pattern resulting from the unique point we are at in history. We are now thirteen thousand years from the last cold and damp epoch of our world's last "Ice Age," more than twice the length of any similar dry period in geological history, and it is doubtful that another cold and damp epoch will occur. Worldwide, we have had thirteen thousand years to "dry out" and, thus, the rampages of these fires. Imperiled by this widespread prevalence of wildfires are entire ecological communities that, for tens of thousands of years, were the accustomed homes of all of our world's native peoples. In my own region, scientists tell us that, as little as seven hundred years ago, one could ride on horseback in pine forest and pine-juniper mixed forest all the way from my Colorado high country to the center of Nebraska or Kansas! This was the landscape that native peoples knew then which has completely vanished today.

So, acting with environmental vigilance today is a part of honoring the very sacred ground of so many native peoples. Such caretaking is a part of Yogic awareness and lifestyle. Having headed two evacuations because of fires within five years, I am now part of a healthy forest initiative involving over 100 acres of my land. In this initiative, we remove selected understory, recreating a stable forest floor of new growth. That supports the endangered older trees, many of which are so old we can see the clear signs of their being wisely pruned by earlier native peoples. We also promise not to sell acreage for money-making "development" which would further impede the natural cycles of the forest's own ability to remain stable and healthy.

Cross-Overs

There are many gratifying mysteries to share here. First of all, I am one of many carriers of Native American traditions who is not, by direct lineage, a Native American. Many of us who have been given a name or responsibilities by Native American leaders, elders, or shamans are often referred to as "adopted" or as "cross-overs." A few years ago, I published an article in *The Contemplative Journal*, along with Dr. Kurt Johnson who has contributed to this book. We shared statistics gathered from publications around the world showing that, in some indigenous teaching traditions, significant percentages of current "lineage holders" or "wisdom keepers" are not of that original "blood lineage" but are from other cultural or ethnic backgrounds. I honor these phenomena as part of the inevitable cosmopolitanization of our planet—our moving toward a one-world culture where the resources of all the wisdom traditions are shared in their abundance. When rightly done, such activity in no way replaces the original integrity of each lineage, nor does it excuse or advocate "misappropriation" of wisdom resources from one group to another. It also does not excuse any lineage's role in the former persecution or annihilation of any other group. It only testifies that we live in a culturally evolving world, a world in which the only answer to complexity is inclusivity, and that inclusivity is, of course, love.

One of the great convergences of our time is that of modern science and the ancient knowledge of our Indigenous peoples—that the Planet Earth is one, interconnected organism. Although millennial to ancient wisdom, the idea was first proposed to science by the British, and later NASA, scientist Dr. James Lovelock. It was further developed, among others, by Dr. Lynn Margulis, a pioneering American scientist also well known as the wife of astronomer Carl Sagan. This "Gaia" view of earth as a superorganism took its name from the Greek goddess of earth.

Since its inception, an entire discipline within academia has arisen around research into Gaia. In fact, there are two schools of scholarship within Gaia Studies. One is called "weak Gaia" where there is a ton of evidence on how interconnected *some* aspects of Mother Earth appear to be. The other is called "strong Gaia" wherein there is a smaller amount of evidence, but accumulating fast, that Gaia is, in fact, an elaborate superorganism. Most recently, the evidence for strong Gaia was enhanced by our knowledge of Plate Tectonics, or Continental Drift, something familiar to nearly everyone today. We used to think of the inanimate (non-living) and animate (living) world as separate. Native peoples never did. We now know, from Plate Tectonics, that the supposedly inanimate world of "rocks" interacts with other aspects of earth—like water and volcanoes—to actually *create* the very gases that allow the origin, and sustenance, of life—oxygen, carbon dioxide, nitrogen, and so on. So, there *is no* separation between animate and inanimate, as our native peoples knew so well.

Again, as with all I have told you in this book about knowledge from the ancients, we see more and more convergence with what modern science also knows is true.

But here is the mystery story I want to share. In the foyer of my house, there resides a large, nearly six-foot tall statue of the revered Eastern deity Quan Yin. Many of you know of Quan Yin I'm sure (also known as Guanyin, Gyan Yin, Kuan Yin, and The Goddess of Mercy), one of the cosmic archetypes and icons of the Divine Feminine. Among my dear friends from the Lakota community is Grand Father White Morning Owl. You'll remember my stories of Fr. Thomas Keating in "Yoga and Sound – Meditation, Manta, and Music." In all the decades of Fr. Keating's now famous work with the Snowmass Inter-religious dialogue, and the creation of the Nine Points of Agreement Among the World's Religions, his main Indigenous colleague was Grand Father Gerald Red Elk. Red

Elk and Morning Owl were contemporaries. As a mystic, Morning Owl experienced visitations from both White Buffalo Calf Woman (the sacred woman and central prophet of the Lakota tradition) and also Quan Yin. Morning Owl was also a gifted painter, so he recorded these visitations in paintings. One day, I showed Morning Owl's painting of Quan Yin to another, prominent, Lakota elder. I was very surprised, in the best way, when that elder said: "I know this depiction is true because you can count in the painting the number of spokes depicted in Quan Yin's halo." I had not even noticed the halo had spokes. The elder continued: "The number of spokes is thirteen—the common number of mainpoles in a Lakota teepee."

As Shakespeare says in *Hamlet*: "And therefore as a stranger give it welcome. There are more things in heaven and earth, Horatio, than are dreamt of in your philosophy."

We are indeed moving toward being One World. Certainly, that is the truest common denominator: one world, one love, one heart. This is certainly the ideal we all seek. It is the ultimate community—the *uni*verse.

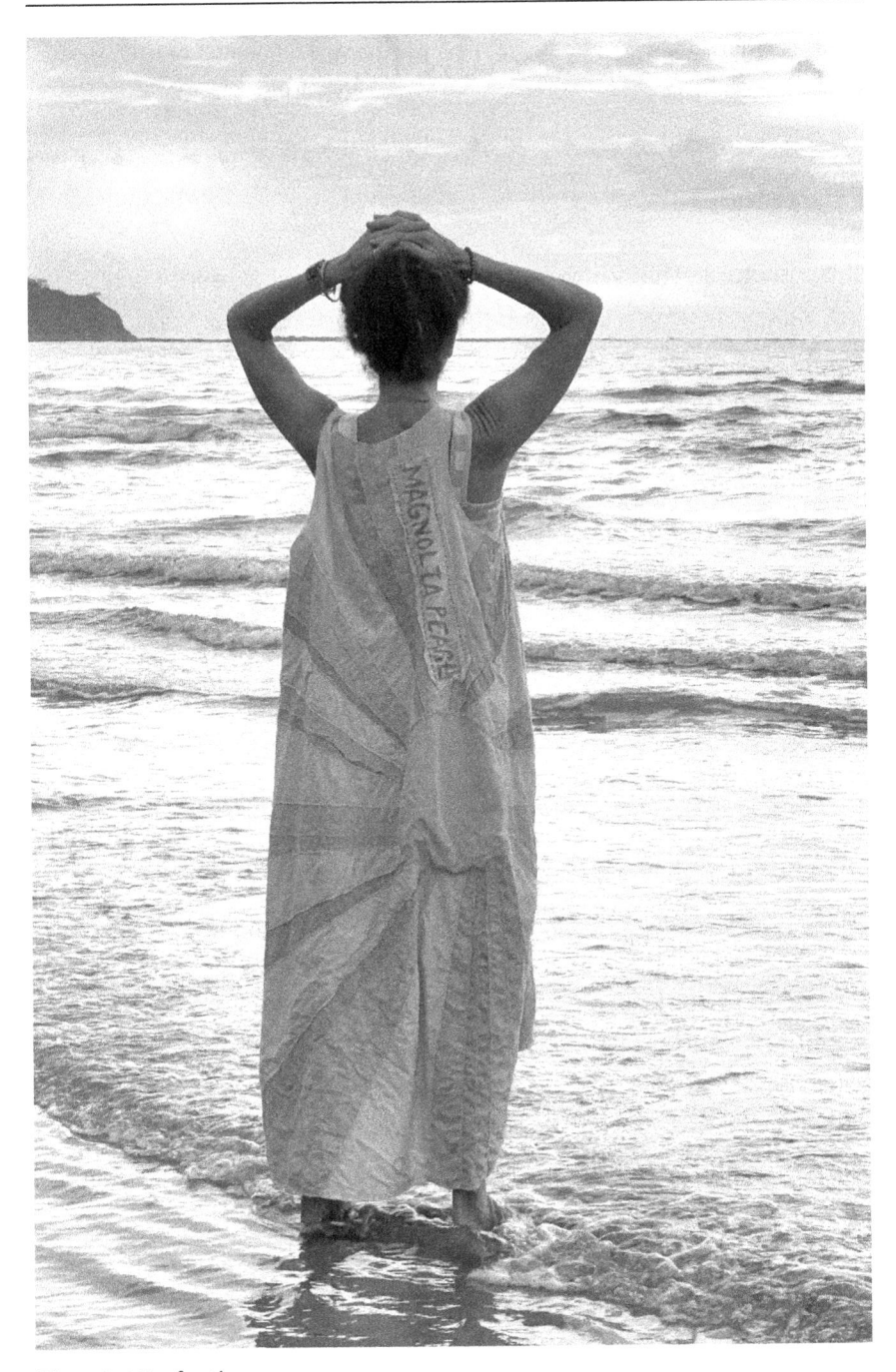

Thou Art Perfection

SHOULD YOU BECOME A TEACHER?

It is inevitable that we would have this discussion, especially when we talk of one world, one heart, one love. As your Yogic voyage continues, you will undoubtedly ask yourself if you might also become a Teacher. If you read Yoga books and websites, you'll see that this question arises to nearly every student, and adept, of Yoga.

There are a number of reasons. First, because you are discovering something so *new*, and so obviously transformative in your own life, it's natural you will want to share it. It's likely you will be so amazed at your own progress, step by step—and all the enhancements of your own health and well-being—that you will start to see the importance of these changes within a bigger, cosmic, landscape—what I called "the Watcher" view earlier in this book. You'll see the incredible value here for yourself and, obviously, for everyone else. From your sense of compassion, you will want all these enhancements to your own life, which often will seem so revolutionary, to also be available for others. Your heart will "kick in," and you'll have this concern about everyone else.

Also on your journey, you will have become aware of the many subtleties, and twists and turns, of the Yogic and Awakening journey. You'll notice how you "almost made *this* decision" or "almost made *that* decision" but "ended up making precisely the *right* decision." That will likely make you ask whether you might be able to offer that kind of deep guidance to others. As well, as I have mentioned before from science, we humans simply like to teach. Contrasting other primates, when we discover something new, we immediately want to share it. This trait truly sets humans apart and has been instrumental in our explosive evolution in technological development. This is kind of "the externals" of it.

With Kundalini Yoga, there are even deeper externals, elements that can move you even more deeply to wonder about your potential role as a Teacher. Kundalini Yoga, as perhaps Yoga's "deepest dive," raises unusual implications for those who may be called to be its Teachers. As you know, Kundalini Yoga is rooted deeply in the mysticisms, and Awakened understandings, of the Great Traditions. Here, it is spoken of as a "Raj" (Royal) Yoga—as a "Direct Path." This does not mean, of course, that other paths are not of equal potential potency and efficacy, not at all. All paths lead to the same place, as Jesus said in the Parable of the Vineyard, shared with you earlier in this book. In fact, one could say that anyone's authentic path is one's *own*, unique, direct path.

However, with Kundalini Yoga's emphasis on the mystical—the deeply devout, the deeply reverent—the authentic call to be a Teacher inevitably brings with it what the Masters call "the deeper depths." This means awarenesses of further and further depth, further nuance, and further sensitivities to subtlety. In this context, you may find yourself "sensing" or "feeling" the call to be a Teacher from a very deep place. It may arise as an insatiable hungering to share—in selfless service—the very elements that have been a part of your own Awakening. In short, in Kundalini Yoga, you may be called to be a "deep feeler." This makes the sense of perhaps being called to be a Teacher in the Kundalini Yoga tradition a very compelling one.

A Deeper Look

What is the calling to be a Teacher, and how does it arise? To understand this, we need to return to Yoga Cosmology and to understandings reflected across all the Great Traditions. What is the "Teacher," and what is the "student, the listener, the learner?"

How does the Teacher/Student serving relationship come about?

Understanding of this is already inherent in the rooting of Kundalini Yoga in the Sikh tradition. The word "Sikh" itself, from the ancient word "*saka*," *means* student, seeker, or disciple. Ultimately, we are all students, and any apparent roles of "Teacher" and "Student" only emerges as an "appearance"–a calling, a role–a dynamic and also a shifting one. It is part of the big cosmic picture of *seva*, of selfless service. Across the vast cosmos, in the great interconnected matrix, "someones" are serving other "someones"–serving "someone's" Awakening. If this is true–and it is–in the bigger picture then, the never changing truth is that we all started in the same place, and we all end up in the same place. So, simply, the "Teacher" is an appearance–a calling, a serving role. After this, when I use the word Teacher and the word student, I always mean it in this context. This way, we can also comprehend what the Great Masters also say: "There is no Teacher. There is no student."

How Does Teacher/ Student Arise?

I'm sure you have heard of the phrase: "When the student is ready, the Teacher appears." This is true. And it is true not just once but many times in our lives–*and* in many contexts–because this is an interconnected universe. You can look back, I'm sure–as I know I can–and remember times (in many settings) where "just the right thing appeared at the right time" or recall when a challenge or trauma appeared that ended up helping guide you rightly on your own unique way. Yes, even during COVID lockdown and social distancing, *still*, so-called Teachers and so-called students found each other by the internet. Within interconnection, as I pointed to just above, there is an *affinity* that exists, indeed already exists, that leads student to Teacher, Teacher to student, friend to friend, and beloved to beloved.

Dogen, the revered Zen Seer, said it this way:

"The student and the teacher are united in affinity, with dharma [their path] and each other."

"In response to affinity the aspiration of Enlightenment arises."

And, perhaps of special significance to us Yogis:

"You will hear it with the body, and you will hear it with the mind."

For the student, this affinity is natural because, as you are proceeding on your Yogic path, your Awakening will also be naturally developing. This is actually why I've chosen the subtitle for this book—"*Your Lifestyle Guide to Yoga and Awakening.*" The centrality of everything for you is your own path, your own Awakening. Its centrality is far deeper than the question of whether you might also be called to be a Teacher. It is, in fact, the well-spring of that calling, should it arise. The central question is about your Awakening. The rest—who is Teacher and who is student—is up to Source. In this context, we can understand the Great Masters' words about Teacher, student, and Awakening.

Once again, from Dogen:

"Endeavor wholeheartedly to follow the path of *earlier sages*."
"Search for that understanding with all-encompassing effort."

Even if:

"You may have to climb mountains and cross oceans."

Or, as in the words from *The Cloud of Unknowing*–

"Even when consumed by the unknown continue with the same all-encompassing hunger for Truth."

Thus, from Dogen:

"The teacher and the student are united in affinity with dharma and with each other. They merge in realization and become one."

This is how we should always understand both the Teacher and the student, how we should always respect the Teacher and the student. It is an affinity, not some kind of achievement. It is the same affinity that we automatically have with Source—Divine to Divine, True Nature to True Nature, True Self to True Self—and, because of this, we always sense the "push-pull" of the relationship, sometimes not knowing which is doing the pushing and which is doing the pulling. Theologians have even figured this one out when they talk about the "ascending energy" and the "descending energy" in our relationship with Source. In that metaphor, we are "reaching up," and Source in "reaching down."

So, if there is a call for you to be a Teacher, it will most likely inherently "arise," and you'll become aware of it. You might be *asked* by a Teacher to become a Teacher, as was my experience, or folks who have become your students—without you knowing it—suddenly point out to you that you are "already" teaching and that you should take it seriously. I know of several cases of very gifted Teachers where it was the eventual Sangha, the circle or community, that actually told *them,* "Hey, you are already teaching, and you should take this calling seriously." That is actually what happened with The Buddha. After his realization under the Bodhi tree, of which I spoke earlier in this book, his friends recognized his newly discovered gifts and apparent freedom and asked that he share this realization with them—that he lead and teach.

Another story can also help us to understand the depth of mystery around the call to be a Teacher and how it unfolds. This is the story of a very famous person, whom I won't name so as not to obscure the real meaning within the story. He is a leader of great stature and has many, many followers. He is one of those persons who is a "reincarnation" of leaders who preceded him. When several of us were sitting with him he shared that many people assume that such "reincarnated ones" are actually "born Awake," but he said this was not true. Such ones, he said, are born with a unique, bountiful, "reservoir of grace" but must, like everyone else, find their own Awakening, and for this, they may need Teachers. The story he told is very endearing and instructive. He said, at first when he was young, he found it strange to have people bowing down to him because he knew "he hadn't figured it out yet." Of course, eventually he did, and he said that, in that process, the Teacher whom he remembered most and to whom he was most grateful was the one who was "hardest" on him. He said of this Teacher, every time I thought "I had found it," he would tell me "No." I would completely think I was on the "right track," and he would tell me "No." Eventually, of course, as it was latent and destined within him, his own Awakening came–and here is the endearing part. He said, "Today, every time I meet that former Teacher in the hallway of the monastery, he winks at me."

Such is the mystery of the inner Teacher and outer Teacher, the Muse of the Divine that flirts with us from behind the latticework, as St. John of the Cross so aptly put it. If the calling is there for you to be a Teacher, it will arise. As one Teacher of mine said, even if you deny it, it will continue to arise.

Just as aptly, one may be as gifted in Awakening as anyone, and yet, one's destiny may be not to teach. Sometimes one's destiny is to just "Be," to, as they say, "leave no traces." Yet, even in those cases, one will likely still end up affecting or helping another person at just the right time for them. In that moment, one becomes the Teacher, just for that situation, and then returns to just Being. A classic writing on the role and kinds of teachers from the Yoga and Vedic traditions speaks of the ephemeral nature of these roles. Some persons *are* called to be Teachers in the traditional sense, and they will do that always, and do it well. Others, Source may call to do just what's right, to be just what's right, at this or that moment for someone. They call that kind of teacher "the Friend."

Ultimately, East or West, recognition of a Teacher, or the calling of a Teacher, has something to do with the identification and choice by an "other," something also universally known as giving sacred "Permission" for the relationship. It can happen at the personal level of Teacher and student as described by Dogen—that mystical relationship—or it can be through recognition by and from a community. Generally, the calling to be a Teacher will always have this collective dimension.

But is this *always* true? Again, the answer is a rare "no," and, again, it's because of the mystical dimension. It might happen that an emerging Teacher is the *only* one who knows his or her calling! In these rare instances, one might feel a calling to do something no one else has done. Initially, even without support of anyone, that called person may simply know "they have to do it." This is rare but there are many historical examples. We know about them because, eventually, they were recognized by a following. Often history moves this way because such emerging leaders are a part of a major movement of shift and change. They are absolute pioneers. You'll remember what I told you about my friend Ken Wilber. He had to strike out on his own, in search of that "theory of everything," and even go around the traditional routes of academic publishing because his message was so new. This is not unique to the spiritual community. There are now-famous scientists who also had to do this; one had to publish his own books, even in a non-English language first, to get the attention his vision deserved. It can happen in many ways.

The Levels of Being a Teacher, and Teacher Responsibility

To return to the externals—in the 3-dimensional world, historically, you will find that the more subtle mysteries about "Teachers" noted above are actually also reflected in how the laws of various nations deal with the recognition of spiritual teachers—that is, of "clergy." It's worth mentioning because there are actual differences between East and West. I mentioned this when I noted how various Ayurvedic practices are "licensed" or their schools "certified" in various nations around the world. This process of required "recognition" is a by-product of the diversity of our planet. Most societies now usually want to reflect diversity, but they also want a sense of order and "quality control." So, when a community rises to the level of needing to form an Ashram, Church, Gurdwara, Synagogue, Mosque, etc. (of which, of course a "Teacher" or "clergyperson" is typically the leader), there are forms to fill out and processes to go through. Universally around the world, the legal forms will ask you how you chose the Teacher, the Pastor, the Rabbi, the Imam, or whatever the case may be! In the West, most traditions have schools they send their eventual clergy to, and they "graduate" and/or are "ordained." In the East, the Teacher is most often "recognized" by the community or is part of a "lineage" from which, traditionally, successful teachers have been drawn—a very different process. One could say that this results from a difference between East and West in that western traditions are more about beliefs (thus the schools and graduating someone who has been "trained") while eastern traditions, whose religions are more centered on consciousness, are more about the more mystical recognition of a Teacher. This is not completely true, however; the western traditions also have their deeply mystical traditions. It's just that they have, historically, less to do with how Teachers are chosen.

When the calling to be a Teacher arises and unfolds, there are also considerations about general protocols and specific ones that accrue tradition to tradition. Kundalini Yoga, because of its mystical dimensions, includes certain specific emphases for a Teacher. From what you have read herein about Sadhana, you will understand why it is believed that the regularity and depth of a Teacher's own Sadhana practice parallels and reflects their effectiveness as a truly serving Teacher. This is because only by their own navigation of all the subtleties of that sacred practice can they have the acumen and gifts to truly and effectively serve those around them.

In Kundalini Yoga, there are also specific publications from the teaching traditions, organizations, and institutions about expected ethics, morals, protocols, and behavior. They generally parallel those for all professional service and therapeutic professions. You will also find many good references and guides, across all the Yoga traditions (particularly the deeper ones well-anchored in the ancient Vedic traditions), about the meaning and responsibilities of the Yoga or spiritual teacher, and I recommend them all. There are also very fine, and important, publications by interfaith, interspiritual, and psychological associations, especially the Association for Spiritual Integrity (spiritual-integrity.org), that well describe diverse aspects of awareness, and right protocols, for the relationship of Teachers and students in the 3rd dimension. The high values in these references and guides are all very important, and my discussion here of the aspects of the deeper dimensions only further supports their insistence on the impeccable ethics and standards required by the role of being a spiritual Teacher. Having all these toolkits available is important since every spiritual teacher of any depth needs to operate successfully on all of these planes.

Companions Forever

The mystery of the role of the Teacher is never ending, rooted in the nature of the never-ending Dharma itself. As Adyashanti is known for saying: "The Truth never changes from the moment you first see it; it only becomes infinitely more refined."

As Dogen said, in the maturing of the Teacher/Student affinity, in consciousness, we will likely forget "who is who" or even where we came from (though we will also have IDs in our wallets!).

The story below about my own mentor, my own original Teacher–Gurmukh Kaur Khalsa–and "me" will illustrate. Recently, she came to visit me. I was telling her about all that had been unfolding, and about this book, and about the whole mystery of how we all mature and inherently move toward our destinies. She looked at me, undoubtedly thinking of all of our years of connection. She said: "What happened? Where did we go? How did we get here?" I mused for a moment and then said: "I think we just needed to grow."

Such a divine Awakening: "Where did we go? How did we get here?" –"We just needed to grow."

Then I said to her, "Thank you so much for mentoring me through that which I would have never, ever, have seen without your mentorship." She replied, "Karuna, you are someone who is very hard not to love. By the teaching and God's grace, we are here, in what I saw as *your* destiny. Remember, you never suggested becoming a teacher. I suggested it. And the minute I suggested it, you were on an airplane."

Yes, from that first airplane ride, I was into seven years of Teacher Training and mentorship–and the paring away of habits, lifestyles, addictions, defenses, arguments, and denials I didn't even know I had. Don't worry, I haven't *not* noticed that my immediately jumping on an airplane at my Teacher's suggestion parallels exactly what I did at the beginning of my modelling career! Nisargadatta Maharaj recounts this description of the interplay of the Divine Self and finite personality. It is, at once, so endearing, insightful, and true about any of us, and our destiny:

"My destiny was to be born a simple man, a humble tradesman with little formal education. My life was of the common kind with desires and fears. Then, through faith in my teacher and obedience to his words, I realized my true being. I left behind my human nature to look after itself until its destiny is exhausted. Occasionally, an old reaction—emotional or mental—happens in the mind, but it is at once noticed and discarded. After all, as long as one is burdened with a personality, one is exposed to its idiosyncrasies and habits.

When I met my guru, he told me, "You are not what you take yourself to be. Find out what you are: watch the sense 'I am,' find your real self." I obeyed him because I trusted him. I did as he told me. All my spare time I would spend looking at myself in silence. And what a difference it made, and how soon. It took me only three years to realize my true nature. My guru died soon after I met him but it made no difference. I remembered what he told me, and persevered. The fruit of it is here with me."

Let us celebrate together the eternal affinity of "Teacher" and "student" and how it mysteriously unfolds for each of us in the service of our own certain Awakening.

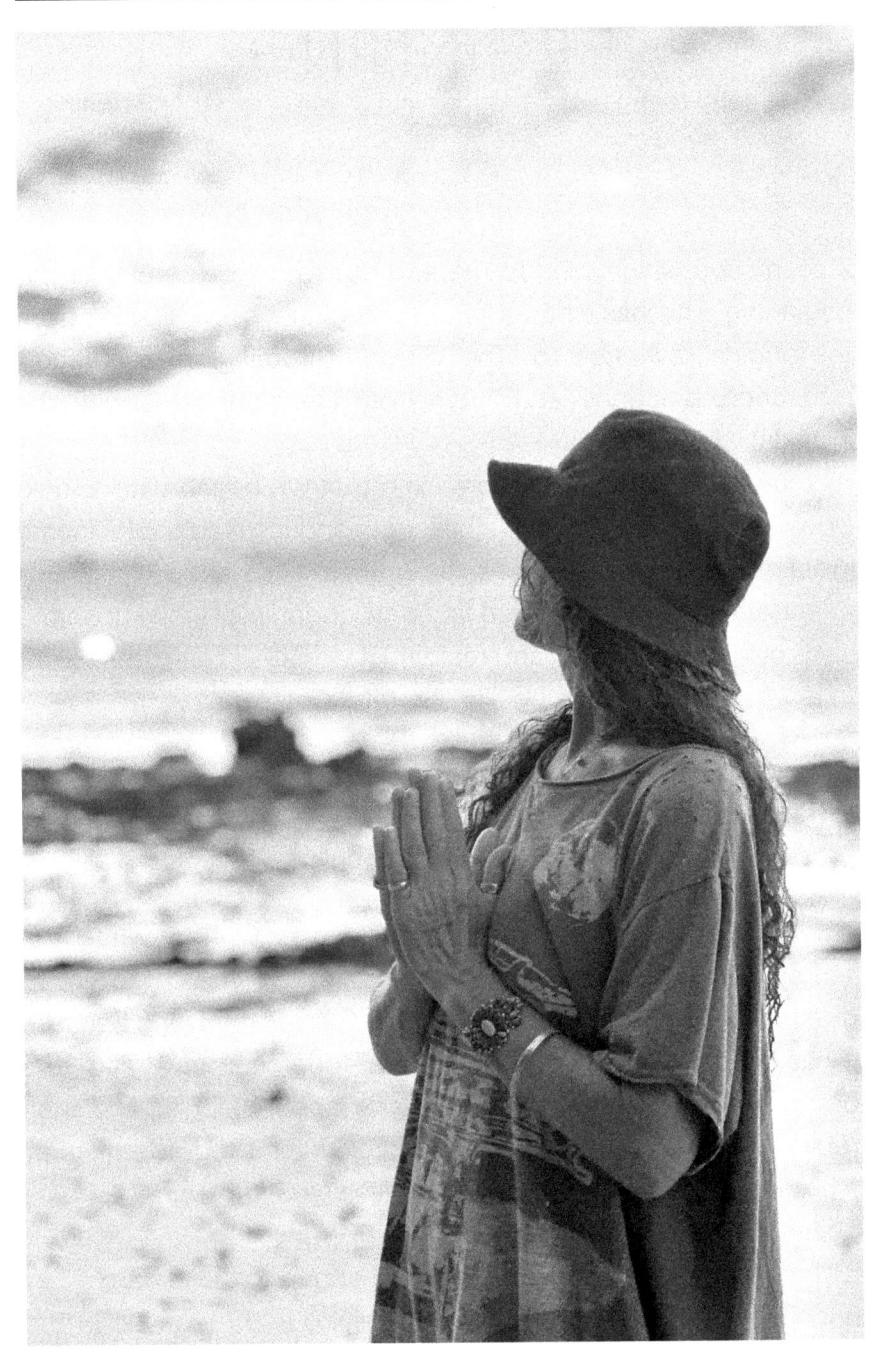

Bhakti Yogi

"ENDING" THIS BEGINNING

It seems we have come to the end of this book—the end of this beginning. This has been a journey we have been sharing from the original invitation to "The Village," through the exploration, inspiration, practices, and setting our life compasses with the incredible gifts of Yoga.

You'll remember at the beginning that we began with "Going Down the Rabbit Hole"—the challenge—and inevitable gifts innate in our consciousness and the birthright in it of authentic Awakening.

You'll remember that Alice (in *her* Wonderland) woke up in the arms of her loving sister, and realizing it was all a dream, they went to tea. In a famous song by "The Grateful Dead" they write:

"And if I awaken you, you may find
that you were dreaming too"...
"it's all a dream we had yesterday—long ago..."

I bring it here because that song was written when the songwriter's father was passing, and he wanted to sing it to him, to give him hope. It has struck many hearts across the world because it has sold millions of copies. So, this—the song, the dream, the book—is, among so many other things, about Healing, and then rebirth and redirection. I hope it has been that for you—a beginning, a healing, and a setting of your course, a setting of your compass points, as I said just above.

The Vedas perennially use the metaphor of the dream. They understand consciousness and Awakening in the context of the levels of the dream—waking consciousness, dream consciousness, and deep sleep, the latter where there is no story, no question of identity, no ups, and no downs. I think we must have deeply known this when we invented amusement park roller coasters. The point is that when we're on a roller coaster we don't think of up as "good" and down as "bad," and when you're finished with one ride, you often get in line and do it again...and then again.

Ending this book, I realized I *must* add that I, too, woke up in the arms of my beloved sister. She was only 21 years old when she passed in a tragic Jeep accident. We were only 15 months apart in age. When we were kids, we shared the same bed. I'm certain we shared the same dreams. Her name was Cathy.

Truly, she is one who has guided me through. She gave me courage and "fight" inside to understand, keep going, and work through my own life, as I have asked *you* to do in this book. We shared all those ups and downs of growing up—schools, friends, foes, being bullied, and all the rest. That close in age, she was my backbone; we leaned on each other for everything, and then she was gone—just like that.

When she passed, I had to make the decision to either stay with my struggling Mom or take a new contract to move to New York City. Here I thank a few very best friends whom I have acknowledged at the end of this book. At that time of my life, much like my helicopter pilot-instructor later, they believed in *my* dream and told me, "Yes, just get on that plane and take off for New York. That's your next step."

Sisters stepped up! I will always cherish them for their bravery and friendship, to point me on my way no matter what shattering happenstances had occurred. It seems I've always had sisters, again and again—and brothers too—the kind of community we have spoken of and lauded in this book and can believe in when life is at its best. These are the people who are the angels in our lives—sleeping or waking, failing or succeeding, and continuing on.

I am so grateful. They saved my life, and they are my angels! I have always been able to trust and breathe again, and I feel this direct communication with my heavenly sister—Cathy—who guided and still does! Connection to the Divine!

The very most I could ask of this book is that it may and could be that kind of an angel, and guide, for you. Remember the wise words of Nisargadatta Maharaj once again:

"When I met my guru, he told me, "You are not what you take yourself to be. Find out what you are: watch the sense 'I am,' find your real self." I obeyed him because I trusted him. I did as he told me. All my spare time I would spend looking at myself in silence. And what a difference it made, and how soon. It took me only three years to realize my true nature."

Well, Nisargadatta was a great seer. As he says, what he did, what he "accomplished," was simply fidelity to his own destiny and birthright. So, as Dogen reminds:

"Endeavor wholeheartedly to follow the path of earlier sages."

My hope, and my assurance actually, is that all of us will follow this simple path, complex as it may seem, and trust that Source will open our route before us. There will be twists and turns. That is part of it, part of the Hero's Journey—the inevitable muddle, and the inevitable resolution. There will be times when it is difficult and dark, truly challenging. There will be times when The Promise—of birthright, of Awakening, of good life—may, as Lao Tsu says, "only seem as if it were there." But, as he says in the very next line, your "use will never drain it."

I trust that life will send you forward from this book with myriad wonderful moments—discoveries, fulfillments, and even ecstasies—perhaps the more unexpected, the better.

So—like Alice and her sister—let's go to tea.

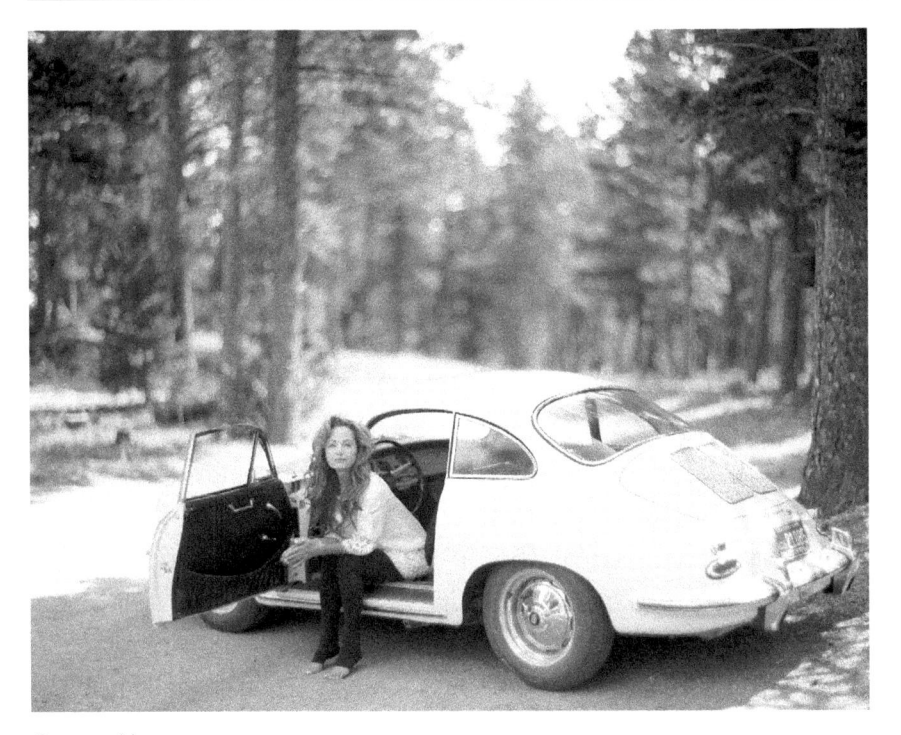

Pepper Her

AFTERWORD

Light on Kundalini: Your Lifestyle Guide to Yoga and Awakening is a beautiful and powerful map to a life of great health, inner peace, and deep spiritual experience.

Yoga, as imparted by the ancient sages, saints, and rishis of the Himalayas, is a comprehensive science and art of well-being. Its history is a rich tapestry, woven over millennia, timeless and boundless in its relevance and applicability. Thus, Yoga is not just about what you do on the mat; it is about how you live your lives. It is about making daily choices that reflect your highest self and your connection to the world around you. Yoga stands as a guiding light, bringing us back into balance with our true Selves, with the Earth, and with each other, mitigating suffering from dis-ease caused by our systems being out of alignment and equilibrium.

This book beautifully bridges the ancient wisdom of Yoga cosmology with our contemporary understanding, showing how the structure of the universe and the dynamics of our own existence are intricately connected. It also dives into teachings around how fundamental qualities of nature influence our human predicament and how we can transcend their grip to find our true birthright of inner peace and freedom. It also shows us our integral oneness with all of Creation—including the animals, the trees, and the rivers. This awareness brings a sense of unity and compassion that extends beyond our personal practice to our interactions with the world.

As you journey through this book and experience its lessons, you will find that Kundalini Yoga is incredibly powerful, guiding you to access, harness, awaken, and work with the very flow of Divine energy within your own bodies. It is available and accessible for all, and the practices are sure to benefit people of all ages, all walks of life, and all levels of experience. The wisdom and practices offered in this book and its companion, *The Light on Kundalini Manual*, compiled from decades of Karuna living, embodying, and teaching Kundalini Yoga, are part of the culmination of her life's mission to guide anyone who is called to undertake this metamorphic journey, illuminating each step with clarity and depth.

At every turn of the page, and twist in the trail, Karuna reminds us that Yoga is a path of transformation. It is a journey of "Self-realization" that leads us to a deeper understanding of who we are and our place in the universe. May this book serve as a compass, companion, and inspiration on your journey of discovery and awakening, and may your Yoga practice help you to find the peace, joy, and love that reside within you and connect you to the divine essence that pervades all of creation.

And whenever you feel called to come home to the birthplace of Yoga in the Himalayas, on the banks of the sacred Mother Ganga river, our arms and doors at Parmarth Niketan are open to you all.

–*Sadhvi Bhagawati Saraswati*
International Director, Parmarth Niketan, Rishikesh
Director, International Yoga Festival
President, Divine Shakti Foundation

YOGA PRACTICE APPENDICES
1-12

Practice Descriptions for the INSPIRED MESSAGES *with Yoga Practices*

Descriptions and explanations below are adapted from Karuna's *Foundational, Day to Day,* and *Sessional Guides in her Yoga Manual.*

1. Foundational Yoga Elements Needed for the Practices in this Book
2. Revisiting the Chakras, with Fuller Details about the Bandhas (or "Locks")
3. Warming Up and Tuning In & Session Closing
4. Our Opportunity to Connect with the Divine
   – *Kriya for Growing Closer to the Divine*
5. Healing Grief
   – *Balancing the Five Tattvas (SaTaNaMa, Kriya for Instinctual Self and Sat Kriya) and Ancient Kriyas for Healing Grief (Pittra Kriya, Shuni Mudra and Superman Pose)*
6. Becoming Zero Over and Over Again
   – *Kriya for Elevation*
7. Awakening the Ten Bodies
   – *Kriya for Awakening the Ten Bodies*
8. Interiors and Exteriors
   – *Balancing with Nabhi Kriya with Prana and Apana*

9. How to Stay Natural
   – *Sat Kriya*
10. Gauging Your Progress and Preventing Burnout
    – *Meditation Against Burnout*
11. Grace and Gracefulness in Transitions
    – *Nahbi Kriya*
12. Recommendations for Recipes and Music

1

FOUNDATIONAL YOGA ELEMENTS NEEDED FOR THE PRACTICES IN THIS BOOK

From Karuna's Yoga Manual, Foundational Guide

In these Yoga Practice Appendices, the instruction "See Foundational Guide" points you to the explanations of this Entry.

Foundational Asanas, Mudras, and Other Elements

For your ease and convenience, descriptions and explanations of asanas, mudras, and other practice elements in these Appendices are adapted from Karuna's Yoga Manual, *Foundational Guide*, *Day to Day Guide*, and *Sessional Guide* and provided below, entry by entry, session by session, as needed. Some of the most universal elements you'll use again and again are directly below; many of them will be described again in the context of a particular practice session.

Warming Up, Tuning In, and Session Closing are explained and described in a separate Appendix 3.

Foundational Sitting Poses

Easy Pose (*Sukhasana*) is the most common sitting position in Yoga, and the position that is most often employed between other position elements (each called an "asana") or sequences of asanas (sequences called "kriyas"). In Easy Pose (often in

English called "sitting cross legged"), you sit comfortably on the ground or floor with your legs crossed in front of you, spine and head straight.

Rock Pose (*Vajrasana*) is a modified version of Easy Pose, often used as part of, or between, other poses as Rock Pose]. You sit as in Easy Pose but, instead of sitting with legs crossed in front of you, the legs are folded under you, and you "sit on your heels."

These are the two most common sitting poses used, or built out from. Other sitting poses will be described individually in the subsequent practice entries, as needed.

Foundational Standing Poses

Mountain Pose (*Tadasana*) is a foundational posture related to all standing poses. You simply stand normally, straight and relaxed, with the feet aligned together, arms hanging comfortably to the side, and with palms open and facing outwards. Mountain Pose is a starting posture for many variations of standing poses which further involve the arms and legs.

Other Standing Poses, some of which are used often in kriya sequences, will be described individually in the subsequent practice entries, as needed.

Foundational Lying (Supine) Poses

Corpse Pose (*Savasana*). This is the most common lying down (supine) pose in Yoga. It refers both to the position itself and also to one of its most universal usages—for resting between or after Yoga Kriyas. In Corpse Pose, one lies prostrate on the back, legs and arms extended outward slightly, as comfortable and with the head relaxed gently, straight, or to the side, as comfortable.

Corpse Pose is often employed between other postures, combined with other movements, or used explicitly for resting (*Savasana*).

Foundational General Body Actions

Sweeping the Auric Field. This is a body movement used with many poses and positions, particularly ones in which one is in a position with the arms/hands raised or extended above the head. It is most often used at the end of an exercise, or asana, to "conclude" the activity. Whether in a standing or sitting position, with the arms/hands raised above the head, one Sweeps the Auric Field by simply bringing down the straightened arms (like wings) to your side, thus "sweeping" the entire field of your aura.

Foundational Breathwork (aka Pranayama–Breath Techniques)

Breathwork in Yoga is often referred to as "the science of breath" because knowledge of breathing in Yogic practice is very exact. Yogic breathing techniques are diverse, ranging from variations of the depth and length of breathing's exhales and inhales (from Simple [or Natural] Breathing to Long Deep Breathing, as below) to more precisely directed techniques (like Breath of Fire, Alternate Nostril Breathing, etc., as also below).

Inhalation and Exhalation. Yogic practice recognizes three regions of the body involved in our capacities for breath-related work: the abdominal area (Abdominal Breath [sit bones to the bottom of the ribs]), the chest area (Chest Breath [bottom of the rib cage to top of the rib cage]), and neck and head area (Clavicular Breath [from the upper rib to base of the skull]). These are treated in much more detail in my *Day to Day Guide*. In the excerpts from my *Foundational Guide*, I will include briefer information on three kinds of breathing that are foundational to most Yogic practice.

Simple (Natural) Breathing. It is important to understand that Simple (Natural) Breathing is not the same as how we may have learned "everyday breathing." Simple (Natural) Breathing begins with inhalation through the nose, with the navel area moving outward, moving air fully into the lungs, and then a full exhale wherein the navel moves in and up, pushing the air fully out. Variations on this regarding frequency, selective holding of the breath, or other details of modality make up the various breathing techniques you will find in Karuna's Manual, *Day to Day Guide*.

Long Deep Breathing. This is a foundational breathing technique used with many Yoga postures (asanas). It expands the length and depth of the breath and utilizes all three of the body's breathing regions (see above under *Inhalation and Exhalation*). It begins with filling the abdominal area, then (by expansion) the chest area, and then the breathing area from the upper rib to base of the skull. Exhalation is the reverse: deflating the upper area, then the chest, and finally the abdomen as it pulls in and up (with the navel moving back toward the spine). The Teacher will prescribe the variations of deep breathing practice including temporary *Suspension of the Breath*.

Breath of Fire (Agni Pran). This is one of the most fundamental breath techniques in yoga. It is used in combination with many other asana postures, and it is important to learn accurately so that it can serve its yogic purposes. Breath of Fire is a rapidly pulsed breathing, from the nose or from the mouth, as instructed—rather like "panting"—which is employable at many different rates. Often, it is learned first by mimicking a dog panting, with the mouth open and the tongue out. As one becomes accustomed to it, it is often advised to learn to do it comfortably, usually by having a strong out-breath which makes the in-breath almost automatic.

Long Deep Breathing (Pranayam option) with Concentration on the Third Eye Point (Ajna point). From the Easy Pose just above, breathe in complete and long breaths while concentrating on the Third Eye Point [with eyes closed, look up at the "Third Eye," the space between the eyebrows, the sixth chakra] for 5 minutes or as instructed by the Teacher.

Nadi Cleansing (Alternate Nostril Breathing). Eye Position: Eyelids can be gently and narrowly open and relaxed, focusing lightly on the Brow Point. Hand Positions (*Mudra*): Thumb and index finger are used to close and open the appropriate nostril ("U-breathing"). Breathing Pattern (inhale, hold, exhale): Holding the right nostril closed with the thumb, inhale through the left nostril; then, opening the right nostril, holding the left nostril with the index finger, exhale through the right nostril. In same position now inhale through the right nostril; then, opening the left nostril, and holding the right nostril with the thumb, exhale through the left nostril. Repeat 3 to 5 minutes or as instructed by the Teacher.

2

REVISITING THE CHAKRAS, WITH FULLER DETAILS ABOUT THE BANDHAS (OR "LOCKS")

Chakras in Yoga Cosmology

The Chakras are listed below in ascending order, including the name in English common usage, their Sanskrit name, the general locations, and the color assigned to the Chakra by the mystical traditions.

1. *Root Chakra ("Muladhara")* – base of the spine (red)
2. *Sacral Chakra ("Svadhisthana")* – just below the navel (orange)
3. *Solar Plexus Chakra ("Manipura")* – stomach area (yellow)
4. *Heart Chakra ("Anahata")* – center of the chest (green)
5. *Throat Chakra ("Vishuddha")* – base of the throat (blue)
6. *Third Eye Chakra ("Ajna")* – forehead, above between the eyes (indigo)
7. *Crown Chakra ("Sahasrara")* – top of the head (violet)

Foundational Knowledge of Bandhas (or "Locks") with Foundational Knowledge of the Chakras

Because the Yoga cosmology of the Chakras is fundamental to Kundalini Yoga, Kundalini practices also requires knowledge of the "Bandhas" (or "*Locks*"). The Bandhas are uses of the muscles in various areas around the spine to channel the energies of Yogic practice, especially the "Kundalini energy." Below, the Bandhas are described in detail, with notes on their primary relationships with the Chakras.

Rootlock ("*Mulbandh*") [pronounced "mool bond"]. Rootlock involves the first, second, and third chakras. It engages the anus and perineum, the sex organs, and the navel point. It aligns the energy to move it up the spine and to circulate the energy generated from this practice. It can be applied with a variety of intensities. The Teacher will advise concerning Rootlock.

In brief here, it works as follows. There are three steps, corresponding to the associated Chakras in ascending order. However, the three steps become nearly simultaneous when this practice is mastered. The three steps are:

For the 1st Chakra: Using your general body senses, gently contract the muscles in the rectal area and anus as if you were holding back a bowel movement; then

For the 2nd Chakra: As if you are withholding urination, gently contract the sex organ area; then

For the 3rd Chakra: With your breath held either in or out, lightly pull the lower abdominal area back toward the spine, pulling the navel area in as you do.

As noted previously, the Teacher will advise further.

Diaphragm Lock ("*Uddiyana Bandha*") [pronounced "oo-di-yana bonda"]. Diaphragm Lock serves the solar plexus and the heart chakra. One begins by exhaling and holding the breath out, then pulling in in the solar plexus, diaphragm, and the muscles of the upper abdomen in towards your spine and then up. Thus, the diaphragm is lifted. This action benefits the heart regions and moves energy up into the various organs of the neck region. The diaphragm is utilized both for Yoga postures and in chanting, as further advised by the Teacher.

Neck Lock or Chin Lock ("*Jalandhara Bandha*") [pronounced "jah-lon-DAR-ah bonda"]. Neck Lock is the most basic and most generally applied lock. It especially serves the throat chakra and, located in the strategic region between the torso and head, is important to all the higher chakras. Neck Lock involves finessed actions and movement wherein the chest and breastbone are moved subtly upward, synchronized with straightening the back of the neck, pulling the chin in, and pulling the head up. When completed, the chin will be resting between the two collar bones while the head is still level, and the vertebrae of the neck are still straight. The shoulders will relax, as will the mouth and tongue. With the aligned, straight, posture across this area, energy can flow freely from the heart center up to the head and brain. The Teacher will advise further regarding Neck Lock.

The Great Lock ("*Maha Bandha*") [pronounced "MAH-ha bonda"]. The Great Lock involves the application of all three of the Bandha ("Locks") nearly simultaneously in a quick sequence, thus providing the results of all the Bandhas at once. Normally, the Root Lock is applied first and, when it is relaxed, the Diaphragm is then applied. When it is relaxed the Neck Lock is then applied and relaxed. The Teacher will further advise on sequences and durations for these applications.

3

WARMING UP AND TUNING IN & SESSION CLOSING

Begin "Warm Up and Tune In" from *Easy Pose*.

Easy Pose (aka *Sitting Cross-Legged, Sukhasana*) is the most common sitting position in Yoga, and the position that is most often employed between other position elements (each called an "asana") or sequences of asanas (sequences called "kriyas"). In Easy Pose (often in English called "sitting cross legged"), you sit comfortably on the ground or floor with your legs crossed in front of you, spine and head straight.

A modified version of Easy Pose, often used as part of, or between, other poses is *Rock Pose* (*Vajrasana*). You sit as in Easy Pose but, instead of sitting with legs crossed in front of you, the legs are folded under you, and you "sit on your heels."

Warming Up

Sitting in *Easy Pose*, hands are drawn together in front of you, palm to palm, and the palms are briskly rubbed back and forth as if to warm them. This livens the arms and body and gets you ready for Yoga practice.

Tuning In

The hands are drawn together, palm to palm, in front of the chest at heart level, as in the gesture of "Namaste" or Eastern bowing. This is also called *Prayer Pose* ("*Pranamasana*") whether done standing or sitting.

In Karuna's tradition, Tune In is done with two short Ancient Chants (mantras) from the Sikh tradition. The language is Gurmukhi, but you'll easily become accustomed to it from the demonstrations and the English transliterations of the words, often used as below.

The opening Mantra is known in the ancient traditions as the *Adi Mantra* (meaning "primal sound"), sometimes colloquially also called simply "*Ong Namo.*" Of course, the Teacher will often demonstrate, but the transliteration below makes it easy:

Ong Namo, Guru Dev Namo
(usually repeated three times, or as instructed)

Pronounced: On "Ong," the emphasis is on the "oNG," letting the NG vibrate in the sinuses and on the upper palate of the mouth. "Namo" is pronounced "Nam" (as in Vietnam) – "O" (oh). Guru is pronounced as in "Gudo." "Dev" is pronounced more like "Dehv."

The literal meaning is usually translated as "I bow to the Creative Wisdom; I bow to the Divine Teacher," meaning, of course, both within and without. This Tuning In connects you to both Source and Self.

This mantra is followed by a second short "mantra of the Heart," also repeated three times or as instructed, and often referred to by its first line: *Aad Guray Nameh*.

Aad Guray Nameh

Pronounced: *Aad* is pronounced more like "odd." *Guray* is pronounced like "gu-ray." *Nameh* is pronounced like "na-meh." This mantra is a prayer for protection and success. Translated through all four of its lines, it means: "I bow to Primal Wisdom; I bow to the Wisdom of the Ages; I bow to True Wisdom; I bow to the great unseen Wisdom." The four lines of the mantra are easily transliterated for English below:

Aad Guray Nameh
Pronounced more like "odd," "gu-ray," "na-meh."

Jugaad Guray Nameh
Pronounced more like "ju-God," "gu-ray," "na-meh."

Sat Guray Nameh
Pronounced more like "sought," "gu-ray," "na-meh."

Siree Guroo Dayvay Nameh
Pronounced more like "Sirie," "Guru," "Day-vay," "na-meh."

After the Tune In, the Teacher then leads the participants into the asanas and kriyas of the session.

Closing a Session

In Kundalini Yoga in the West, sessions end with the song "Long Time Sun" and then two or more sung "Long Sat Nam" as lead by the Teacher.

Closing Song
"Long Time Sun"

May the long time sun
Shine upon you
All love surround you
And the pure light
Within you
Guide your way on
Guide your way on
May the long time sun
Shine upon you

All love surround you
And the pure light
Within you
Guide your way on
Guide your way on

4

OUR OPPORTUNITY TO CONNECT WITH THE DIVINE

— with Kriya for Growing Closer to the Divine

Kriya for Growing Closer to the Divine

Introduction from Karuna

This Kriya invites us to grow closer to the Divine—and that is all of us and all things! This is Divine Community! To join with All, let's grow closer to our daily practice and meditation, and also freer from distractive noise—inside and out. This kriya intentionally emphasizes the meditative—quieting and calming. With appropriate asanas for the body, it moves through breathing, cleansing, and mindfulness—and then culminates in a deep resting with gong and mantra. With daily awareness, we are realizing and finding Peace, Harmony, and the Creative Forces within and around us. True Community! Many blessings from my Heart to yours!

Kriya Sequence

Begin with *Tuning In* [see Yoga Practice Appendix 3]. Then follow this sequence (1-9).

1. *Sufi Grind* (*Siri Om*) (3 minutes as instructed by the Teacher) Beginning in *Easy Pose* [see Yoga Practice Appendix 1], grasp the kneecaps with the hands and rotate the torso in circles, holding the head nearly stationary. Use the spine like a "grinding wheel," going first clockwise numerous times and then

counterclockwise numerous times, etc. as further instructed by the Teacher.

2. *Bowing* (*Dhanurasana*) (3 minutes as instructed by the Teacher)
Generally, bowing can be seated or standing, moving or still (the Teacher specifies). From *Easy Pose / Prayer Pose* [see Yoga Practice Appendices, Entry 1], do repeated slow and reverent waist bows, breathing as appropriate.

3. *Knee Bounce* (*Butterfly Knees*) (2 minutes as instructed by the Teacher)
From the *Easy Pose* just above, beginning gently, bounce the knees up and down, becoming more vigorous as possible (be cautious and measured regarding vigor if you have any chronic knee complaints). As you bounce the knees, inhale and exhale deeply in a rhythm that suits you.

4. *Long Deep Breathing* (*Pranayam option*) (5 minutes as instructed by the Teacher)
From the *Easy Pose* just above, breathe in complete and long breaths while concentrating on the Third Eye Point (Ajna point) [with eyes closed, look up at the "Third Eye," the space between the eyebrows, the sixth chakra].

    Note: In this kriya "Growing Closer to the Divine," Karuna asks that, while practicing this asana, you "scan the body for tensions and pain" and "relieve these by 'equalizing'–consciously relaxing those areas."

5. *Nadi Cleansing* (*Alternate Nostril Breathing*) (3 to 5 minutes as instructed by the Teacher)
Eye Position: Eyelids can be gently and narrowly open and relaxed, focusing lightly on the Brow Point.

    Hand Positions (Mudra): Thumb and index finger are used to close and open the appropriate nostril ("U-breathing").

    Breathing Pattern (inhale, hold, exhale): Holding the right nostril closed with the thumb, inhale through the left nostril;

then, opening the right nostril, holding the left nostril with the index finger, exhale through the right nostril.

In same position, now inhale through the right nostril; then, opening the left nostril, and holding the right nostril with the thumb, exhale through the left nostril. Repeat, or as instructed by the Teacher.

6. *Front Life Nerve Stretch* (*Paschimottanasana* or *Siri Om*) (90 seconds as instructed by the Teacher)

   Front Life Nerve Stretch is combined with a breathing asana "inhale, head up" and "exhale, head down." Take slow but powerful breaths, increasing speed as instructed by the Teacher (be careful not to compress the neck when moving the head back).

   Life Nerve Stretch Variations can also involve, on the exhale: (1) alternate bending of the back and head toward the knees, reaching out with the arms and hands to touch the toes, first right, then left, or (2) bending of the back and head toward the center, reaching out straight with the arms and hands between the legs. The Teacher will instruct concerning these choices and the number of repetitions.

7. *Breath of Fire* while in *Corpse Pose* (3.5 minutes as instructed by the Teacher)

   Perform *Breath of Fire* (see Yoga Practice Appendix 1) and *Corpse Pose* (see "How to do Savasana" below, under Nabhi Kriya, Entry 11).

   In "Growing Closer to the Divine," Karuna asks that, while practicing Breath of Fire from Corpse Pose, you also shake/move your body, as motivated in the moment, to "expel pain" and "negativity." Consciously concentrate on these expulsions as you do this asana.

8. *Savasana*

   See "How to do Savasana" below, under Nabhi Kriya, (Yoga Practice Appendix 11).

In "Growing Closer to the Divine," Karuna also would like to invite you to experience her gong with her in her sacred space, which you may find in this video with Yogi Amandeep Singh on her Light on Kundalini YouTube channel at:
https://youtu.be/2CokzYALKbE?si=vQMNd8MSsX9hiVh8

9. *Seated Meditation with Mantra ("The One Meditation")*
In "Growing Closer to the Divine," Karuna ends the Kriya with 15 minutes of the Mantra "God and Me, Me and God, are One" from *Easy Pose* [see Yoga Practice Appendices, Entry 1] sitting with palms up and hands in *Gyan Mudra* [see Yoga Practice Appendices, Entry 5].

While the mantra is sung, the right hand is moved step by step from chakra to chakra, starting from the base of the spine to the crown chakra above the head. After each stepwise movement, the hand drops slowly from the crown to the base of the spine, and the sequence is repeated.

A good rendition of this Mantra can be found at:
https://mantradownload.com/en/products/me-and-god-are-one-yogi-bhajan

5

HEALING GRIEF

– Balancing the Five Tattvas (SaTaNaMa, Kriya for Instinctual Self and Sat Kriya) and Ancient Kriyas for Healing Grief (Pittra Kriya, Shuni Mudra and Superman Pose)

Reconcile, Rejuvenate, Heal, and Awaken to the Light of Your True Self

Kundalini Yoga, known as "the Yoga of awareness," is an ancient technology for awakening the life force lying dormant within each one of us. Conceptualized as a sleeping serpent, coiled up at the base of our spine, this latent source of primordial energy is mobilized through the actions and components of the kriyas that lie at the heart of Kundalini Yoga practice.

A Kriya is a sequence of physical movements or postures that often include pranayam (breathwork), mantras (sacred syllables), mudras (hand positions), bandhas (body locks), as well as eye focus and angular positions to awaken, direct, and contain the flow of this spiritual energy within.

Join Karuna as she leads you through powerful ancient Yoga practices known for their deeply spiritual, meditational, and subtle-realm elements. Karuna demonstrates and explains the wisdom of each to help you explore the depth of your grief and heal it.

Grief is the first layer of trauma. We store grief under our anger, resentment, destruction, and the way we speak to ourselves. It's important to understand the layers of grief so we can release them.

Healing Grief Practice

Healing Grief Practice is divided into three convenient modules that include inspiration, wisdom message, Yoga practice, self-reflection, journaling, and rest and relaxation. They can be done sequentially or in individual sessions. Begin each session, if they are practiced separately, by "Warming Up and Tuning In," and end each session with "Session Closing" (See Yoga Practice Appendix 3).

Module 1: Getting the Body Out of Distress

Grief, anxiety, worry, fear, concern, etc. are not just experiences in our psyches and emotions. Because we are holistic organisms of spirit and body, all psychic and emotional elements are also deeply embedded in our bodies.

In Healing Grief, it is important first to make the body comfortable by knowing that it is recognized and loved, thus calming and relaxing the body and creating the environment for a whole-systems approach to the transformation process we are undertaking. This is one of the great gifts of Yoga.

Getting the Body Out of Distress Practice

Begin session with "Warming Up and Tuning In" (see Yoga Practice Appendix 3), then proceed.

The flow sequence for this Kriya includes the following flowing elements. Karuna will guide the duration and flow of these 18 elements which Karuna will instruct. The elements include: Thigh Slap, Knee Massage, Calf Pound, Knee Massage, Thigh Pound, Legs Apart, Kundalini Spiral, Hip Raises, Shoulder Pound, Chest Slap, Forehead Tap, Spine Rolls, Snake Hips, Rest, Cat Stretch, Neck Lift, Rest, and Self Massage.

The first four elements (Thigh Slap, Knee Massage, Calf Pound,

Knee Massage) begin from *Modified Easy Pose*, which is *Easy Pose* simply modified to have the legs stretched out in front of you. Easy Pose is the most common sitting position in Yoga, and the position that is most often employed between other position elements (each called an "asana") or sequences of asanas (sequences called "kriyas"). In Easy Pose (often in English called "sitting cross-legged"), you sit comfortably on the ground or floor with your legs crossed in front of you, spine and head straight.

Then, for the next two (Thigh Pound and Legs Apart), the legs are spread apart as in moving into *Life Nerve Stretch* (*Paschimottanasana* or *Siri Om*). Be seated with your legs stretched out and spread wide in front of you. Inhale, sitting with your spine straight (or as straight as possible). Grasp each big toe (or, if can't, some location closer to you–foot, ankle, etc.), keeping the back as straight as possible. Life Nerve Stretch can then involve, on the exhale: (1) alternate bending of the back and head toward the knees, reaching out with the arms and hands to touch the toes, first right, then left, or (2) bending of the back and head toward the center, reaching out straight with the arms and hands between the legs. The Teacher will instruct concerning these choices and the number of repetitions.

Kundalini Spiral begins from *Easy Pose* (see above).

Hip Raises, Shoulder Pound, Chest Slap, and Forehead Tap *begin* from *Corpse Pose*. This is the most common lying down pose in Yoga. One lies prostrate on the back, legs and arms extended outward slightly as comfortable, and the head is relaxed gently, straight or to the side, as comfortable. As in this case, Corpse Pose is often employed between other postures, combined with other movements, or used explicitly for resting (*Savasana*).

For Spine Rolls / Back (Spine) Rolls, begin in Corpse Pose (above) as instructed by the Teacher. Pull the knees into the chest with the front of the face between the knees, as comfortable. Then rock/roll back and forth, rolling on the spine or as instructed by The Teacher.

For Snake Hips, *rest* from lying position, Corpse Pose (see above) as instructed by Karuna.

Cat Stretch begins in Corpse Pose (see above).

Begin in Corpse Pose (above) and follow Karuna's directions for Neck Lifts.

Rest (*Savasana*) in Corpse Pose (above).

Self Massage from Easy Pose (above) as instructed by Karuna.

Module 2: Balancing the Five Tattvas

Ancient wisdom discovered five qualities of our senses in the world and our senses of the world. After quieting and relaxing the body, we want to balance these five essential ways that we all sense in, and of, the world.

The ancient traditions called these "Earth, Water, Fire, Air, and Ether." Today, we know ether as Consciousness and the intertwining of earth, air, fire, and water as the essential "states of matter"—gases, liquids, and solids—and their combustions (fire) that have formed both our bodies and the entire universe.

These Kriyas are ancient ones nurturing this balance.

Sa Ta Na Ma Kriya
Kriya for Instinctual Self
Sat Kriya

1. **Sa Ta Na Ma Kriya**

    Begin session with "Warming Up and Tuning In" (Yoga Practice Appendices, Entry 3), then proceed.

    Sit in *Easy Pose* (above) with a straight spine, and a light *Neck Lock* (Yoga Practice Appendix 2).

    Place your wrists on your knees, with the arms straight, start with hands in *Gyan Mudra (Gesture of Consciousness or Seal of Knowledge)*. Gyan Mudra is perhaps the most well-known mudra to public parlance. The hand is held open, palms up, with the tip of the thumb joining with the tip of the index finger (to form a circle). Gyan Mudra has two variations—active and passive. In "active," the index finger is tucked under the end of the thumb; in "passive," the tips of the thumb and index finger are touching directly. The passive version is the most widely used.

    Focus your eyes at the tip of the nose.

    Make an 'O' shape with your mouth. Breathe in long and slow as you mentally chant "Saa Taa Naa Maa," and repeat as you breathe out. You must hear the hissing sound of the breath going in and out through the 'O' shape of the mouth. With each silent repetition of the sound, alternate between four mudras:

    On Saa, press the thumb and index (Jupiter) fingers together.
    On Taa, press the thumb and middle (Saturn) fingers together.
    On Naa, press the thumb and ring (Sun) fingers together.
    On Maa, press the thumb and pinkie (Mercury) fingers together.

    To End the Kriya:

    Inhale deeply. Make a fist of your hand by placing the thumb of the mound of Mercury and folding the fingers down over the thumb. Squeeze the fist tight, squeeze the whole body tight, and hold the breath for 15 seconds. Cannon fire the breath out.

Inhale deeply again and hold the breath for 15 seconds. Tighten your fists and squeeze the whole body. Let the energy spread to every muscle. Use Cannon Fire breath on the outbreath.

Inhale very deeply for the last time and hold for 15 seconds. Gather the whole universe of your muscles, and everything you have. Squeeze from the toes to the top of your head. Let it go and relax.

2. **Kriya for the Instinctual Self**

   Begin session with "Warming Up and Tuning In" (Yoga Practice Appendix 3), then proceed.

   The flow sequence for this Kriya includes the following elements: Butterfly Pose, Cobra Pose, Crow Pose, Leg Lifts, Modified Boat, Relaxation Rock, Shoulder Stand, Plow Pose, Sat Kriya from Celibate Pose, and Relaxation (Savasana).

   Butterfly and *Butterfly Bends* (*Badhakonasana* or *Titli Asana*). Beginning in Easy Pose (see Foundational Guide) bring the soles of the feet together while grasping the feet with your fingers; spine and head should be straight. Begin by bouncing the knees up and down, with the level of vigor instructed by the Teacher. Butterfly is often combined with bends, such as (1) similar to spinal flex, on the inhale arching the spine forward and lifting the chest, and then, on the exhale, arching the spine backward or (2) rotating the vertical spine and head, or bending it left and right, as instructed by the Teacher.

   Cobra Pose. Lie prone on the floor with palms flat on the floor under the shoulders. As you inhale, arch the spine up slowly, leading with first the nose, then the chin, and finally pushing off and up with your hands, progressing vertebra by vertebra until you are arched back as far as possible but with no strain in the lower back. Concentrate on a comfortable stretch from the heart center upward. Breath modality can depend on instruction of the Teacher, either breathing deep and long, or accompanying the exercise with *Breath of Fire* (for *Breath of Fire*, see Foundational Guide).

Crow Pose. To come into Crow Pose from standing, squat down and place your hands flat on your mat about shoulder-width apart with the fingers spread wide. Now, keep the hands and feet where they are but lift the hips way up toward the sky, bend the knees and lift the heels off the floor so just the balls of the feet are down.

Leg Lifts–Back Reclining Leg Lifts. For these leg lifts, you will be lying on your back with your arms stretched along your side. Then, or as instructed by the Teacher, with legs straight, the legs are then lifted to 30-, 60-, or 90-degree angles (and held) or moved through these positions as a "sweep." Inhale as you are raising the legs; exhale as you are lowering them. If done as a "sweep," keep raising and lowering the legs, letting your breath lead the movement. The teacher will instruct further regarding duration and breathing. For individual exercise, if done as a "sweep," one to three minutes is usually normative.

Modified Boat. Follow instructions by Karuna from *Boat Pose*. Begin seated with your knees bent and feet flat on the floor, hands resting beside your hips. Keeping your spine straight, lean back slightly and lift your feet, bringing your shins parallel to the floor. Draw in your low back, lift your chest, and lengthen the front of your torso.

Relaxation Rock. Follow instructions from Karuna.

Shoulder Stand (*Salamba Sarvangasana*). In this pose's final position, you will be resting on your shoulders, neck, and back of the head while your torso and extended [straight] legs will be perpendicular and extended in a straight line toward the ceiling.

You begin by lying supine on your back with legs extended and arms at the side. Inhaling, use the abdominal muscles to lift your legs and hips off the floor, followed by curling your torso in and bringing the knees toward your face. Continuing, lift the hips to bring your torso perpendicular to the floor, using your arms for support by bending your elbows (elbows aligned parallel with the body) and placing your hands (fingers pointing up) on your buttocks/torso to provide support. Finally, from this position, you can lift your thighs so they are vertical to the floor, and following, when ready, bringing your legs and feet vertical as well, pointing toward the ceiling. As you attain this completed position, all of your body will naturally adjust to comfortably holding this pose, with your head and neck comfortably in line with the spine, gazing toward the chest and not turning the head to the side.

The Teacher will instruct as to duration. In individual practice, the pose can be held for 10-15 breaths for starters, and up to five minutes or longer in experienced yogis.

You can exit Shoulder Stands or work from it to other poses by a number of options. You can gently lower the straightened legs above your head, into Plow Pose; you can gently lower the buttocks and torso, by slowly removing the support of the arms and returning to either Fish Pose, or lying prone again on your back.

Plow Pose (*Halasana*). In this pose's final position, you will be resting on the back of your shoulders with your arms stretched out straight along your side (to steady you) so that the legs can be lifted up and over your head to touch the toes to the floor above your shoulders and head.

One moves into this pose sequentially as below, usually starting from *Shoulder Stand* (*Sarvangasana*) since from

Shoulder Stand the only remaining action to complete Plow Pose is, upon exhale, bending from the hips to slowly lower your toes to the floor above and beyond your head. When this is done, the torso should be perpendicular to the floor, the neck and head flush with the mat, and the legs fully stretched and extended. You will notice that the outstretched arms along your torso will naturally steady you and adjust accordingly. To exit Plow Pose, bring your hands to steady your torso and, on exhalation, gently lift the legs up into Shoulder Stand once again; then, on a later exhalation, you can simply roll down onto your full back again and be out of both poses.

3. **Sat Kriya**

   Begin session with "Warming Up and Tuning In" (Yoga Practice Appendix 3), then proceed.

   In Sat Kriya, you will combine a sitting position with a positioning of the joined and parallel outstretched, straight, arms moving up and down in a "pistoning" position. This motion is accompanied by a verbal chant of "Sat" and "Nam" as explained further below.

   Begin in *Celibate Pose* [aka *Hero Pose*, "*Virasana*"]. This is a famous classical sitting pose across all the Yogas. It differs from the other sitting poses in that one sits "*between* the feet," the lower legs being placed on each side of the hips. This contrasts *Easy Pose* [sitting simple cross-legged], the three various cross-legged sitting poses noted just above, and *Rock Pose* [sitting on the heels].

   The outstretched, straight, and interlaced arms are then to be moved upwards and downwards, outstretched from you, as you chant, repetitively "Sat Nam," with "Sat" on the upward movement and "Nam" on the downward movement. You will note that "Sat" will pull in the navel, while "Nam" will relax the navel.

   End the Kriya with Relaxation (*Savasana*) in *Corpse Pose*, which is the most common lying down (supine) pose in Yoga. It refers both to the position itself and also to one of its most universal usages—for resting between or after Yoga Kriyas. In Corpse Pose, one lies prostrate on the back, legs and arms extended outward slightly, as comfortable, with the head relaxed gently, straight or to the side, as comfortable.

Module 3: Ancient Kriyas for Healing Grief

Pittra has an ancient history in the East for healing from calamity, grief, or disaster. The word itself means "ancestor" or "history" and, thus, directly refers to something lost.

Ancient Kriyas for grief like those in this module were often practiced in nature, especially by a river, to give the sense of healing with the flowing of time.

In Yoga, stress is seen as a "frozen" state. It needs to be released with relaxation of both body and spirit, which is the function of these three Kriyas.

Pittra Kriya
Shuni Mudra
Superman Pose

1. **Pittra Kriya**

    Begin session with "Warming Up and Tuning In" (Yoga Practice Appendix 3), then proceed.

    The left hand rests on the Heart Center with the right hand cupped in front of you. Elbows are relaxed at your side.

    Eyes are focused on the tip of the nose.

    The right hand reaches up and passes the ear as if you are splashing water over your shoulder. Feel the wind pass the ears as the hands move toward the shoulder. The wrist must cross the earlobes; the hand must travel that far back.

    To end, stretch the hand back as far as you can and suspend the breath for 15 seconds.

Exhale.

Repeat two more times.

2. **Shuni Mudra**

    Begin session with "Warming Up and Tuning In" (Yoga Practice Appendix 3), then proceed.

    Place the elbows on the second rib, below the base of the breast, in line with the nipple.

    Hands are slightly wider than the elbows, and the palms are facing up in *Shuni Mudra* —the thumb covers the nail of the middle (Saturn) finger.

    Eyes are focused at the tip of the nose.

    As you repeat "Har," flick the Saturn finger, as demonstrated by Karuna.

    To end, inhale deeply, continuing to move the fingers.

    Suspend the breath for 15 seconds, letting it open the rib cage, balancing the Chakras.

    Do a Cannon Breath exhaled, as instructed by Karuna.

    Repeat three times.

3. **Super Man Pose**

    Begin session with "Warming Up and Tuning In" (Yoga Practice Appendices, Entry 3), then proceed.

    Bring the arms out in front of you in a "V," about 15 degrees above shoulder height–in Superman Pose. Hands are flat and facing down.

    At a rate of one repetition per second, repeat "Har" as in the second exercise, crossing the hands in front of you and keeping the arms straight. Don't bend the elbows.

    Alternate crossing one hand over another.

    To end, keep moving the arms and inhale for 10 seconds, breathing out with Cannon Breath (as instructed by Karuna).

    Repeat 3 more times, moving the hands as fast as possible in the last repetition.

6

BECOMING ZERO OVER AND OVER AGAIN
– with The Kriya for Elevation

Kriya for Elevation

This is a classic Kriya from the Kundalini Yoga tradition which is also comfortable for practitioners of all levels and practiced always in the traditional sequence below.

Introduction from Karuna

This *Kriya for Elevation* is one that anyone at any stage of their lives, whether 7 or 80 years old, can do. It's a systematic set of exercises that are an excellent tune up. They help aid the circulation of the breath, in and out, and the body's energies moving up and down the spine. With each step–from *Ego Eradicator* (which exercises and opens your lungs and brings alertness to the brain) to the movement *Spinal Twists* (to rotate left and right, balancing the hemispheres of the brain), to *Front Life Nerve Stretch* (which involves the legs, slow breath, and lengthening of the spine, and even grasping your toes, if you can)–this Kriya stretches the body. Then, as you bow forward in a deep experience of honoring *yourself*, you taste a truly devotional Yoga. The Kriya then reaches to the Heart, opening you further with the "hood of courage"–*Cobra Pose* ["*cour*" meaning Heart!]. Finally, you lie on your belly to rest, soaking in Mother Earth and culminate by waking back up to enter into the intense and impactful movement of *Sat Kriya*. This is one of Kundalini Yoga's most effective Kriyas for elevation and rebirth.

We as a community sometimes stop listening as we keep on leaping. Now is the time to start weeping—and the weeping comes from the vulnerable place of "I Bow," "I Bow into this New Awakening."

Kriya Sequence

Begin with "Tuning In" [see Yoga Practice Appendix 3]. Then follow this sequence (1 - 11).

1. *Ego Eradicator* with *Breath of Fire* (for 1-3 minutes as instructed by the Teacher).
   For the *Ego Eradicator* asana, begin in *Easy Pose* [Simple "Sitting Cross-legged" or "Indian Style," see Foundational Guide]. Then close your fingers, curling the fingertips to the top pads of your palm (like a fist) but with the thumbs extended "up and away." Then, lift your arms, keeping them straight, to a 60-degree angle. The thumbs of your curled fist will thus be aimed generally at each other from both sides of your head. This pose, as "Ego Eradicator," is usually combined with *Breath of Fire* (see Foundational Elements in Yoga Practice Appendix 1), holding the pose, with eyes closed and adding the breath. The Teacher will advise regarding duration and details for breathing. For individual exercise, the duration is usually 1-3 minutes. To end Ego Eradicator, inhale and, with arms straight, bring the thumbs to touch, above your head. Exhale as you open the fingers and *Sweep the Auric Field* [see Foundational Guide].
2. *Spinal Flex* (for 1-3 minutes as instructed by the Teacher).
   For the *Rock Pose* asana begin in *Easy Pose* [see Foundational Guide]. With both hands, grasp the ankles and inhale deeply, while arching the spine forward and lifting the chest. Then exhale, arching the spine backward. Spinal flex is usually done

with deep rhythmic breaths. The Teacher may suggest chant-related words to accompany each of these actions (for instance, in Kundalini Yoga, "Sat" on the inhale, and "Nam" on the exhale).
3. Spinal Twists (for 1-3 minutes as instructed by the Teacher).
For *Seated Spinal Twist* asana in this kriya begin in *Easy Pose* [see Foundational Guide]. Raising the elbows high, with arms paralleling the floor, grasp your shoulders with thumb to the back and fingers to the front. Then, on inhale, twist the torso and head to the left. Then, on the exhale, twist to the right. Continue back and forth, ending with an inhale facing straight, and then exhaling to end the sequence and relax.
4. *Front Life Nerve Stretch* (for 1-3 minutes as instructed by the Teacher).
In this Kriya, *Front Life Nerve Stretch* is combined with a breathing asana "inhale, head up" and "exhale, head down." Be seated with your legs stretched out and spread wide in front of you. Inhale, sitting with your spine straight (or as straight as possible). Bending forward, grasp each big toe (or, if you can't, some location closer to you–foot, ankle, etc.), keeping the back as straight as possible. Then bend the back and head further forward, reaching out straight with the arms and hands between the legs, and eventually dropping the elbows so that the head can reach as low to the legs as possible (be careful not to compress the neck when moving the head back). Then return the torso and head upward again. Do this in sequences of "inhale up," "exhale down."
5. *Modified Maha Mudra* with *Breath of Fire* (for 1-3 minutes as instructed by the Teacher).
Begin sitting with torso straight and both legs stretched out in front of you. Beginning with the right leg, bend it inward toward you, reaching out and grasping the right foot, so that you can pull it into the crotch and tuck it inside, heel comfortably against,

or even under, your buttock. Tuck in the chin and put your gaze toward the extended big toe; then reach out with both arms, bending forward with torso and head, and grasp that toe, foot, or shin (depending on your level of comfort). The "work" of the posture is to hold this position for an advised period of time, return to sitting up, and then re-assume the posture, but this time with tucking under the alternate leg. This *Modified Maha Mudra* is as above, except that while holding the fully bowed, completed, pose, one does *Breath of Fire* [see Foundational Guide] for 1-3 minutes. This is repeated, of course, for each switching of sides [right, left, etc.] in assuming the pose.

6. *Life Nerve Stretch to Alternate Knees* and then *Forward* (for 1-2 minutes, and 1 minute respectively, as instructed by the Teacher).

   Be seated with your legs stretched out and spread wide in front of you. Inhale, sitting with your spine straight (or as straight as possible). Grasp each big toe (or, if you can't, some location closer to you–foot, ankle, etc.), keeping the back as straight as possible. On the exhale, bend the back and head toward the right knee, touching the right knee with the head as much as possible (arms and hands still reach out to both toes). Then return upward and repeat this motion of torso and head to the left knee. Alternate the sequence for 1-2 minutes. Finally, on returning upward and to the center, while still with arms extended and grasping the toes, bend the back and head toward the center, touching the head toward the floor as much as possible. Repeat this forward bend for 1 minute or as instructed by the Teacher.

7. *Cobra Pose* with *Breath of Fire* (for 1-3 minutes as instructed by the Teacher).

   Begin lying prone on the floor with palms flat on the floor under the shoulders. As you inhale, arch the spine up slowly, leading first with the nose, then the chin, and finally pushing off and up with your hands, progressing vertebra by vertebra until you are arched back as far as possible but with no strain in the lower back. Concentrate on a comfortable stretch from the heart center upward. In this Kriya, when the back is arched in full *Cobra Pose* commence *Breath of Fire* [see Foundational Guide] for 1-3 minutes as instructed by the Teacher. To complete the asana, inhale and arch the back as much as possible, then exhale, apply *Rootlock* [*Mulbandh*] [see Foundational Guide], and inhale once again. Then exhale slowly, exiting the pose and lowering yourself to the floor to relax for a while, as instructed by the Teacher.

8. Shoulder Shrugs (for 1-2 minutes as instructed by the Teacher).
Rising out of your resting prone position, sit in *Easy Pose* [see Foundational Guide] once again. Then, in an alternating rhythm, shrug both shoulders up on the inhale, down on the exhale or as further instructed by the Teacher.

9. Neck Rolls (for 1-2 minutes as instructed by the Teacher).
Again, sitting in *Easy Pose* [see Foundational Guide], keep the spine straight but relaxed. By slightly moving the head back and bringing the chin down slightly, position the head so that it feels like it is sitting on top of the spine. Then roll the neck slowly in one direction, and then the other direction, letting the head's weight move the head about. Do this slowly and attentively to work through areas of tightness or tension. The Teacher will instruct concerning the number of repetitions.

10. *Sat Kriya* (for 3-7 minutes as instructed by the Teacher).
In *Sat Kriya*, you will combine a sitting position with the joined and parallel outstretched, straight, arms moving up and down in a "pistoning" position. This motion is accompanied by a verbal chant of "Sat" and "Nam" as explained further below.

Begin in *Rock Pose* [see Foundational Guide], that is, in sitting position, legs bent underneath you and "sitting on your heels."

Stretch your arms over your head with elbows straight, right aside the ears. The hands grasp each other, with the fingers interlaced, except for the index finger which is kept pointed straight. Men should then cross the right thumb over the left, while women cross the left thumb over the right.

The outstretched, straight, and interlaced arms are then to be moved upwards and downwards, outstretched from you, as you chant, repetitively "Sat Nam," with "Sat" on the upward movement and "Nam" on the downward movement. You will note that "Sat" will pull in the navel, while "Nam" will relax the navel.

11. Relax in *Easy Pose* [see Foundational Guide].

Completion Message and Direction from Karuna

Take a deep inhale. Focus on the first Chakra right at the base of the spine where *Mata Kundalini* lives. Allow her to awaken inside of you that most profound place of authentic voice, sincerity, strength, and courage, sitting right in you, dormant through many lifetimes. It's time to wake her up. Then, move right up those Chakras—to the 2nd, 3rd, 4th, 5th, 6th, and 7th. Place an intention for *how* you can allow this awakening of *Mata Kundalini*, from 1st to 7th chakra, as this *Kriya for Elevation* has re-elevated you, changed your brain, and given you this opportunity to Awaken. It is *You*, your action that is needed to chant the *Sat* on inhale and *Nam* on exhale, empathetically to yourself, and in a constant rhythm as you move *Mata Kundalini* energy through each of these chakras.

7

AWAKENING THE TEN BODIES
– with Kriya for Awakening the Ten Bodies

Nurture your direct experience with your Soul Body, Negative Mind, Positive Mind, Neutral Mind, Physical Body, Arcline, Auric Body, Pranic Body, Subtle Body, and Radiant Body with Kundalini Yoga.

Kundalini Yoga, known as "the Yoga of awareness," is an ancient technology for awakening the life force lying dormant within each one of us. Conceptualized as a sleeping serpent, coiled up at the base of our spine, this latent source of primordial energy is mobilized through the actions and components of the kriyas that lie at the heart of Kundalini Yoga practice.

Yoga cosmology recognizes ten "bodies" that every human possesses and expresses. One might best consider these as ten capacities or varieties of experience and expression that are a part of our understanding as human beings. Millennia of Yoga practice has shown that each of these ten bodies is very real in experience and can be tended to, and nurtured, by specific Yoga practices.

Link for Free Online Instruction

You can be led through this session by Karuna, free of charge, through her "Awakening the Ten Bodies" program online at Sacred U and Humanity's Stream:

https://courses.sacredstories.com/courses/tenbodies

https://stream.humanitysteam.org/awakening-the-ten-bodies-with-karuna

She leads you through these powerful poses and explains the wisdom. The asana descriptions below are from Karuna's Instructional Guides, step by step. This also helps you familiarize yourself with standard Instructional Guide formats Karuna uses.

Awakening the Ten Bodies Elements

(1) Stretch Pose—with Breath of Fire; (2) Nose to Knees with Breath of Fire; (3) Ego Eradicator; (4) Life Nerve Stretch; (5) Spinal Flex (Camel Ride); (6) Spinal Twists; (7) Arm Pumps; (8) Alternate Shoulder Shrugs from Easy Pose; (9) Neck Turns or Rolls; (10) Frog Pose; (11) Laya Yoga Meditation; (12) Spinal Flex from Easy Pose; (13) Spinal Flex from Rock Pose; (14) Spinal Twist; (15) Bear Grip with See Saw Elbows; (16) Spinal Flex from Easy Pose; (17) Shoulder Shrugs; (18) Neck Rolls; (19) Bear Grip with Locks; (20) Sat Kriya; (21) Savasana.

Kriya Sequence

1. *Stretch Pose—with Breath of Fire*
   Stretch Pose is a lying down pose, on your back with the head, legs, and arms then raised and held, as may be variously instructed by the Teacher. It is often combined with various options regarding breathing, in this case *Breath of Fire* (see Foundational Guide).

   For the basic pose, extend your legs outward in front of you, with your arms resting at your sides. Then move into the Stretch Pose by raising the head, arms and legs as follows, rather simultaneously: lengthen the back of your neck and lift your upper chest, head, and arms off the ground, drawing your chin in. Direct both your fingers and your gaze toward your toes.

The lower back should be flat against the floor. Then lift the legs 6 inches off the floor, toes pointed. If this is difficult or causes back pain, you can further support yourself by keeping the heels slightly resting on the ground and/or placing your hands underneath your sacrum (or sit bones). The Teacher will advise regarding duration and breathing. Often this pose is combined with Breath of Fire (see Foundational Guide).

2. *Nose to Knees—with Breath of Fire*

    Nose to Knees is a variation of *Knees to Chest* in which, after assuming Knees to Chest pose (below), you place the nose between the knees and do *Breath of Fire* (see Foundational Guide) for 1-3 minutes as advised by the Teacher.

    Knees to Chest (aka *Supine Knees-to-Chest Pose*). In this pose, lying on your back, you will have rolled up your knees so that your bent legs are tucked into your chest. Begin supine on the back with arms and legs extended in line with your body. On exhale, simultaneously draw both of your knees to your chest, placing your arms around them. As you do, keep your back as flat on the mat as possible. Depending on your flexibility and comfort, you may be able to grasp the elbows of the opposite arms with your hands. Your body will naturally adjust to this posture with your chin slightly tucked and with your line of sight into your tucked legs.

    The Teacher will instruct as to duration and variations. In individual practice, holding the pose for up to 1 minute, breathing normally, is normative. One often used variation is to, once in this position, gently roll the back forward and backward, or side to side, as if to massage the back (see *Back Rolls*). You can exit the pose by simply releasing and extending both legs again outward in a straight line with the body. In individual practice, assuming and releasing this pose is often repeated up to six times.

3. *Ego Eradicator*
   Ego Eradicator. Sit in *Easy Pose* (see Foundational Guide). Then close your fingers, curling the fingertips to the top pads of your palm (like a fist) but with the thumbs extended "up and away." Then lift your arms, keeping them straight, to a 60-degree angle. The thumbs of your curled fist will thus be aimed generally at each other from both sides of your head. This pose, as "Ego Eradicator," is usually combined with *Breath of Fire* (see Foundational Guide), holding the pose, with eyes closed and adding the breath. The Teacher will advise regarding duration and details for breathing. For individual exercise, the duration is usually 1-3 minutes. To end Ego Eradicator, inhale and, with arms straight, bring the thumbs to touch, above your head. Exhale as you open the fingers and *Sweep the Auric Field* (see Foundational Guide).
4. *Life Nerve Stretch*
   Life Nerve Stretch (*Paschimottanasana* or *Siri Om*). Be seated with your legs stretched out and spread wide in front of you. Inhale, sitting with your spine straight (or as straight as possible). Grasp each big toe (or, if you can't, some location closer to you—foot, ankle, etc.), keeping the back as straight as possible. Life Nerve Stretch can then involve, on the exhale: (1) alternate bending of the back and head toward the knees, reaching out with the arms and hands to touch the toes, first right, then left, or (2) bending of the back and head toward the center, reaching out straight with the arms and hands between the legs. The Teacher will instruct concerning these choices and the number of repetitions.
5. *Spinal Flex (Camel Ride)*
   Spinal Flex (aka *Camel Ride*). Sit in *Easy Pose* or *Rock Pose* as instructed by the Teacher (for Easy Pose and Rock Pose, see Foundational Guide). With both hands, grasp the ankles

and inhale deeply, while arching the spine forward and lifting the chest. Then exhale, arching the spine backward. In some traditions, the Teacher may suggest chant-related words to accompany each of these actions (for instance, in Kundalini Yoga, "Sat" on the inhale, and "Nam" on the exhale). The Teacher informs concerning the number of repetitions.

6. *Spinal Twists*

    Full Seated Spinal Twist. Begin seated with the legs extended out in front of you and your hands rested on your thighs. Bending the right knee, cross the right leg over your left leg and plant the foot next to the left thigh. Then bend that left leg back alongside your right buttock so the right ankle rests comfortably along the right buttock (if this part of the sequence is uncomfortable for you, or as advised by the Teacher, you can use the *Half* or *Modified* version). Now you are in position to twist the torso as follows: wrap your left arm around the top of the right knees and place the right arm stretching downward along your side touching the hand to the mat. From these positions of the left arm on the right knee, and the right arm steadying you from the mat, you will be comfortably twisting the torso. You can increase the twist by bending the left arm and placing the left elbow inside your right knee. This completes the sequence for leading with the right leg and knee.

    The sequence is then repeated, only leading with the alternate, left limbs, as sequenced above. Relaxing the pose or moving into the twists is done with each exhale and inhale, exhaling as you twist. You exit the pose by simply returning to the seated position, legs stretched out in front of you and ready to move into the next sequence.

7. *Arm Pumps*

    Sitting in *Rock Pose* (see Foundational Guide) with arms in front of you, interlace the fingers ("Venus Grip") and hold arms straight. Then, alternately, on the inhale, stretch the arms with interlaced fingers up over your head, and, on the exhale, bring the arms down again to your lap. Duration is 1-3 Minutes or as instructed by the Teacher.

8. *Alternate Shoulder Shrugs from Easy Pose*
   Shoulder Shrugs. Sit in *Easy Pose* or *Rock Pose* (see Foundational Guide) as instructed by the Teacher. Shrug both shoulders up on the inhale, down on the exhale or as further instructed by the Teacher. Duration of 1-2 minutes is normative for individual exercise.

9. *Neck Turns*
   Sitting in *Easy Pose* (see Foundational Guide), keep the spine straight but relaxed. By slightly moving the head back and bringing the chin down slightly, position the head so that it feels like it is sitting on top of the spine. Then, as if saying "Yes" and "No," on the inhale turn your head to the left, and on the exhale turn your head to the right. Do this for 1 minute. Then reverse the sequence, turning your head right on the inhale and left on the exhale for 1 minute. Continue the sequence as instructed by the Teacher.

10. *Frog Pose*
    Frog Pose and *Frog Pose Variations* [*upward facing, downward facing*] [aka *Mandukasana*, or modified as *Bhekasana*, etc.]. This is a squatting posture much like you're "sitting like a frog"—thus the name. The pose is combined with various movement and breathing options as will be instructed by the Teacher.

    You come into *Frog Pose* by "getting down on all fours" with the arms stretched out in front of you and with your legs spread open and flat on the floor, heels thus aimed up, and the feet thus "pointing toward each other." Yes, much like a frog! Variations on the pose then involve *"upward facing"* (head and upper chest/shoulder arched up, arms thus used to push up and/or hold), or "*downward facing*" (head and upper chest aimed down, or even on the floor, as the Teacher may instruct, with arms either straight out in front of you, or bent in support at the elbows, as the Teacher may instruct). Movement in and from Frog Pose involves pushing up or down, and/ or in repetitions from upward facing to downward facing combined with inhaling up and exhaling down with a strong and steady rhythm of the breath. The Teacher will advise regarding duration, repetitions, and breath. For individual exercise, repetitions may range from "best effort" to 26 or 54 repetitions, the latter two being the common numbers of repetitions usually prescribed.

11. *Laya Yoga Meditation*

    Begin in *Easy Pose* (see Foundational Guide) with hands in *Gyan Mudra* [see Yoga Practice Appendix 5], placed on the knees. Chant in sequence, as further instructed by the Teacher: *Ek Ong Kaar-**uh**! Sa Ta Na **Ma**! Siree Wha-**uh**! Hay Guroo!* On each **emphasis**, firmly lift the diaphragm; relax it on *Hay Guroo*. Visualize the energy moving up your spine on each sequence. Continue sequencing for 11 minutes, or 31 minutes, depending on instruction from the Teacher.

12. *Spinal Flex from Easy Pose* (see 5, above)
13. *Spinal Flex from Rock Pose* (see 5, above)
14. *Spinal Twists* (see 6, above)
15. *Bear Grip with See Saw Elbows*

    In *Bear Grip*, the fingers are closed on each hand and then opened slightly to lock them together, each hand pulling the opposite direction. In *Sea Saw Elbows*, the arms, in Bear Grip, are raised in front of you and rocked diagonally up and down, with the elbows alternatively extending up toward the ear and down to the side.

16. *Spinal Flex from Easy Pose* (see 5, above)
17. *Shoulder Shrugs* (see 8, above)

18. *Neck Rolls*

    Sitting in *Easy Pose* [see Foundational Guide], keep the spine straight but relaxed. By slightly moving the head back and bringing the chin down slightly, position the head so that it feels like it is sitting on top of the spine. Roll the neck slowly to the right 5 times, and then 5 times slowly to the left; inhale and straighten the neck. Continue the sequence as instructed by the Teacher.

19. *Bear Grip with Locks* (see 15, above, and Locks instruction from the Teacher)

20. *Sat Kriya*

    In *Sat Kriya*, you will combine a sitting position with joined and parallel outstretched, straight, arms moving up and down in a "pistoning" position. This motion is accompanied by a verbal chant of "Sat" and "Nam" as explained further below.

    Begin in *Rock Pose* (see Foundational Guide), that is, in sitting position, legs bent underneath you and "sitting on your heels." Stretch your arms over your head with elbows straight, right aside the ears. The hands grasp each other, with the fingers interlaced, except for the index finger which is kept pointed straight. Men should then cross the right thumb over the left, while women cross the left thumb over the right.

    The outstretched, straight, and interlaced arms are then to be moved upwards and downwards, outstretched from you, as you chant "Sat Nam" repetitively, with "Sat" on the upward movement and "Nam" on the downward movement. You will note that "Sat" will pull in the navel, while "Nam" will relax the navel.

    The Teacher will advise regarding durations and repetitions, which can range from 3-31 minutes. Sat Kriya is often used in kriya commitments for daily practice for periods like 40 days, or others, to achieve certain desired results. The Teacher can further advise.

21. *Savasana*

Corpse Pose (*Savasana*). This is the most common lying down (supine) pose in Yoga. It refers both to the position itself and also to one of its most universal usages—for resting between or after Yoga Kriyas. In Corpse Pose, one lies prostrate on the back, legs and arms extended outward slightly, as comfortable, and with the head relaxed gently, straight or to the side, as comfortable.

Corpse Pose is often employed between other postures, combined with other movements, or used explicitly for resting (Savasana).

8

INTERIORS AND EXTERIORS
– Balancing, with Nabhi Kriya with Prana and Apana

A Kriya for Balancing, The Nabhi Kriya for Prana-Apana

Prana and *Apana* refer, respectively, to the physiological "intake" and "output" of our bodies (our intake of food and liquid; the output of our waste products of excretion, menstruation, and so on). Thus, the balanced movement of *Prana* and *Apana* are fundamental to the healthy "life force" of our bodies [see the Ayurvedic sections of the book].

This Kriya begins with focus on the navel point region and the nuances of the Third Chakra, and then moves upward to nurture the body's Heart Center.

The Kriya is always practiced in the classic sequence below.

Introduction from Karuna

We are contemporary Yogis. We need order to balance our day-to-day tasks with our personal Yoga practices. This is a powerful way to cultivate the balance of *prana* and *apana*– "in" and "out" –through breath. These energies are essential to fundamentally balancing our self service, our householder responsibilities, and our lifestyle. Life*cycle* is all about our changes, and that all stems from inhale and exhale. That's our world of change, and it changes on every inhale and exhale. If that isn't exquisite, I don't know what is.

Because the energy of activity is flow, its central locations involve the lungs, the heart, and our digestive systems. We all know that if our digestive tract is "off" we immediately experience "dis"-ease. Our conscious actions with breathing can bring the rebalancing needed, and this is what the natural intelligence of *prana* and *apana* is all about. Even if we just learn to inhale and exhale longer, we can actually eliminate stress buildup, viral residue, and assist a healthy digestive process.

I often use a count for my breath in my personal practice. It's fun to see if I can inhale, hold, and exhale, each for 30 seconds. Even 20 seconds, or just 10 or 5 seconds, will have a health dividend. Try it! Be patient, of course, and build up little by little. Use your active awareness to see the value of your progress! Watch how fast you'll see a transformation. Remember, it's *you* doing the Yoga of Awareness. This Yoga works, immediately, and that's why I love it.

Trust! Believe in yourself and have faith. Lose the fears that block you from enjoying. When you live in fear you stop breathing, and when you stop breathing you start reacting. So, *Prana* is your friend! We are *Pranayee*. We are called *Pranayee* because we are breathing beings. This is what will dissolve distrust and fear. It also makes us more patient.

Kriya Sequence

Begin with "Tuning In" [see Yoga Practice Appendix 3]. Then follow this sequence:

1. *Life Nerve Stretch Variation* with *Breath of Fire* (1-2 minutes, change legs 1-2 minutes, as instructed by the Teacher)
   Be seated with your right leg stretched out in front of you and the left foot on your right thigh, sitting with your spine straight (or as straight as possible). Then grasp the big toe of your right foot with both hands, with thumbs on the big toes and the first

two fingers on the softer areas of the toes. Pulling back on the big toes, straighten the back as much as possible. Apply *Neck Lock* [*Jalandhara Bandha*] (see Yoga Practice Appendix 2) and do *Breath of Fire* (see Yoga Practice Appendix1) for 1-2 minutes as instructed by The Teacher. Then inhale and change legs, again doing Breath of Fire for 1-2 minutes as instructed by The Teacher. Inhale and then relax.

2. *Kicking Buttocks* (1-3 minutes as instructed by the Teacher)
Begin lying on your back in *Knees to Chest* pose (see Yoga Practice Appendix 7). After assuming Knees to Chest, drop the arms to your sides, palms down, and then lightly begin alternately kicking the buttocks with the heels, inhaling as each leg is raised, and exhaling as it kicks the buttocks. This can be continued for 1-3 minutes, as instructed by the Teacher.

3. *Leg Pistoning* (1-3 minutes as instructed by the Teacher)
Beginning on the back, raise the legs about a foot and a half. Draw the left knee to the chest with an inhale. Re-extend the left leg as you exhale, keeping it elevated while you draw the right knee to the chest. Continue to alternate the legs in this piston-like motion (not bicycle), with powerful breathing, as instructed by the Teacher. Continue 1-3 minutes, as instructed by the Teacher, and end by extending both legs and resting and relaxing.

4. *Front Platform* with *Breath of Fire* (1-3 minutes as instructed by the Teacher)
Front Platform looks much like the "up" position of a push up. Begin by lying prone on the stomach. Bringing your arms upwards with a bend in the elbows, and hands with palms flat on the mat, and arching your feet and leading from the tucking of the toes (as you move the arms and legs to do a conventional "push up"), bring the body up off the floor, keeping the body in this straight alignment, along with the head which will be

looking at the floor. In this position, the angle formed by your body with the floor will be about 30 degrees. Then begin *Breath of Fire* [see Foundational Guide] for 1-3 minutes as instructed by the Teacher.

5. *Stretch Pose* (Pose and Breathing as instructed by the Teacher) This is a lying down pose, lying on the back with the head, legs, and arms then raised and held, as may be variously instructed by the Teacher. It is often combined with various options regarding breathing.

   For the basic pose, extend your legs outward in front of you, with your arms resting at your sides. Then move into the *Stretch Pose* by raising head, arms, and legs as follows, rather simultaneously: lengthen the back of your neck and lift your upper chest, head, and arms off the ground, drawing your chin in. Direct both your fingers and your gaze towards your toes. The lower back should be flat against the floor. Then lift the legs 6 inches off the floor, toes pointed. If this is difficult or causes back pain, you can further support yourself by keeping the heels slightly resting on the ground and/or placing your hands underneath your sacrum (or sit bones). The Teacher will advise regarding duration and breathing. Often this pose is combined with *Breath of Fire* (see Foundational Guide).

6.-10. Heart Center Stretch for Healing

For this sequence, follow these seamless elements:

6. Begin sitting in *Easy Pose* (see Foundational Guide). Then stretch your arms fully from your sides, fingers extended, thumbs up, as if you were surprised to see someone and greeting them. Breathe deeply a few times in this position. Then clench your fists, strongly, and in sweeping, forceful, motion bring the fists strongly to your chest, exhaling forcefully as you do. Repeat this

outstretched and "to your chest" strong movement of the arms 2 or 3 times as instructed by the Teacher.
7. Then stretch the arms out again as above, stretching also the fingers and thumbs, and hold them there strongly for 1 minute.
8. Then slowly bring the arms back toward the chest but, this time, ending with the palms of the hand facing each other in front of your chest about 4 inches apart. Hold this pose, while gazing into the space between the hands, for 1-2 minutes as instructed by the Teacher.
9. Then bring the hands together in front of the chest in *Prayer Pose* and meditate quietly, to the *Brow Point*, for 1 minute.
10. With the hands still in *Prayer Pose*, do a *Sitting Front Bend*, bending the torso and forehead to the floor, and relax in this position for 1 minute.
11. Return to sitting up in *Easy Pose*. Guided Meditation by the Teacher.
12. Relaxation as instructed by the Teacher.

Completion Message from Karuna

This is one of the most moving, wildly inventive, Yogic practices I have ever encountered. I never imagined something like this, so fiercely capturing, could offer me this type of Awakening and awareness, courage and grit, and stamina and vitality. This is what these Kriyas and Meditations bring—it is so incredibly wondrous. Ultimately, I am so hopeful that this work will change your life, to become your life, as it has mine.

9

HOW TO STAY NATURAL
– with *Sat Kriya*

Sat Kriya

Practiced from a single sitting Yoga pose, *Sat Kriya* is a classic Kriya that is one of the most powerful and often used Yoga Kriyas.

Introduction from Karuna

I give Sat Kriya to anyone who wants to change. Because it stimulates the natural flow of energy, it strengthens the character—inside and out—and it relaxes you to control your behaviors just enough that you can catch them when you are in the middle of them and ask, "Is this what I still want to be?"

Dance, joy, happiness! Live serenity and grace. These 11 minutes a day will give you a creative flow that you can't help but *dance*. Let the Spirit dance. Let the Spirit dance—barefoot, with the drum of your heart and the sound of the birds singing in the sight of the butterfly dancing in you!

Kriya Sequence

Begin with "Tuning In" [see Yoga Practice Appendix 3]. Then follow this sequence.

In *Sat Kriya*, you will combine a sitting position with joined and parallel outstretched, straight, arms moving up and down in a "pistoning" position. If instructed, this motion can be accompanied by a verbal chant of "Sat" and "Nam" as explained further below.

Begin in *Rock Pose* [see Foundational Guide], that is, in sitting position, legs bent underneath you and "sitting on your heels." Stretch your arms over your head with elbows straight, right aside the ears. The hands grasp each other, with the fingers interlaced, except for the index finger which is kept pointed straight. Men should then cross the right thumb over the left, while women cross the left thumb over the right.

The outstretched, straight, and interlaced arms are then to be moved upwards and downwards, outstretched from you, as you chant "Sat Nam" repetitively, with "Sat" on the upward movement and "Nam" on the downward movement. You will note that "Sat" will pull in the navel, while "Nam" will relax the navel.

The Teacher will advise regarding durations and repetitions, which can range from 3-31 minutes. Sat Kriya is often used in kriya commitments for daily practice for periods like 40 days, or others, to achieve certain desired results. The Teacher can further advise.

To end the sequence, as instructed by the Teacher, inhale and apply *Rootlock* ("*Mulbandh*") [see Yoga Practice Appendices, Entry 2] concentrating on the movement of the energies up and down your spine. Exhale and apply *The Great Lock (Maha Bandha)* [see Yoga Practice Appendix 2]. Then inhale and relax.

Completion Message from Karuna

When you chant "*Sat*" on the inhale, feel the energy wave all the way from the tailbone to the Crown Chakra and exhale, sending it right back to the center of the Ocean. In each action of Sat Kriya, see it as this dynamism of drawing from, and giving back, to the Divine Ocean. What is also important about Sat Kriya is for you to lay out, at the end, for the same amount of time that you have put into the overt external actions of the Kriya. This is very important because the real work comes *after*, believe it or not! When you are doing the overt external work, you are "pumping it up." It is the time after when the real balancing of the energies in your body takes root.

10

GAUGING YOUR PROGRESS AND PREVENTING BURNOUT
– with Meditation Against Burnout

Meditation Against Burnout

Begin with "Tuning In" [see Yoga Practice Appendices, Entry 3] if you have not done so already as part of a larger sequence.

This practice is most effective when it can be done with plenty of time, especially to relax and be quiet after completing it.

Begin in *Easy Pose* [see Foundational Guide] with the spine straight.

The hand positions (Mudra) are important, as they create a state of dormant energy which assists in the modes of relaxation and quiet.

Raise the arms with elbows bent such that the two forearms are quite in a straight, or slightly inclined, line with each other and so that the *backs* of your palms meet each other and are held touching each other; the fingers are then dropped/pointed down and the thumbs crossed over the inside of the hands, near touching the ring (Mercury) ring finger.

In this position, keep the arms and hands in place but also comfortable and relaxed.

Then focus the eyes on the tip of the nose.

Deeply inhale through the nose in eight equal and sequential intakes. Then completely exhale in eight equal and sequential outbreaths. If you like, the pace of the in and out breaths can be synchronized with thinking "Sa Ta Na Ma, Sa Ta Na, Ma."

Initial practice session should be done for 11 minutes. It can then be enhanced to a 22-minute session and then a 31-minute session.

11

GRACE AND GRACEFULNESS IN TRANSITIONS
– with Nabhi Kriya

Nabhi Kriya

Nabhi Kriya is another classic Kriya from the Kundalini Yoga tradition. "Nabhi" refers to the nerve matrix around our navel point and the region of the 3rd Chakra. The 3rd Chakra, also known as *Manipura* or "lustrous gem" Chakra, is related to the energies of empowerment, self-confidence, self-knowledge, and our transformative and "warrior" energies.

Introduction from Karuna

Put a smile on your face as you do this Kriya and ask yourselves: "Am I ready for this? Am I already living this?" You might already be there, I'm guessing. So, ask yourselves what brought you here today, to this amazing Nabhi Kriya to strengthen the core of your being, in exactly the right timing for you. It is the only way we can call you, and the only way you can answer. The answers are with you. So, follow Nabhi Kriya precisely and watch for any urges you have to "switch it up" or change it. If you need to make adjustments, to decrease this or that element, be sure to do so consistently. You can decrease the demands of this Kriya but remember that the positive effects of the Kriya will work for you best if you make such adjustments consistently across the sequence.

What do we mean by "gut brain," and what is sitting there? Ask yourselves, "What is sitting in my gut right now?" Can you swallow fear, grief, and chaos and move into light? Can you allow the miracle of God, and Guru, to be your life? Can your inner environment reflect the world of blue sky above and vibrant, green, mineral-rich soil below, with animals running and funning about in health and delight? Happy, healthy, holy gut! Do you have the guts to go on?

Kriya Sequence

Begin with "Tuning In" [see Yoga Practice Appendices, Entry 3]. Then follow this sequence (1-7).

1. *Alternate Leg Lifts* (for 10 minutes as instructed by the Teacher)
   Begin, lying on your back. Slowly inhale, pulling the lower belly in and lifting the left leg to 90 degrees; point the toes toward the ceiling. Then lower it, exhaling as you do. If needed for support, the hands can be placed on the hips. The leg lifts are then alternated for the duration of the exercise. You then move immediately to the next exercise.

2. *Leg Lifts* (for 5 minutes as instructed by the Teacher)
   Lie on your back with the arms raised straight and stretched, positioned perpendicular to your torso, with open palms touching. Then lift both legs, in straight, sweeping, motion to perpendicular, 90 degrees, to your body. Go back and forth, as in a "sweep," from legs lowered to legs perpendicular, inhaling as you are raising the legs, and exhaling as you are lowering them. In this "sweep," keep raising and lowering the legs, letting your breath lead the movement. Then move to the next exercise.

3. *Knees to Chest* (for 5 minutes as instructed by the Teacher)
   Lying on your back, roll up your knees so that your bent legs are tucked into your chest. On exhale, simultaneously draw both of your knees to your chest, placing your arms around them as

you do and keeping your back as flat on the mat as possible. Depending on your flexibility and comfort, you may be able to grasp the elbows of the opposite arms with your hands. Your body will naturally adjust to this posture with your chin slightly tucked and with your line of sight into your tucked legs. Use this position as a *Resting Position* for 5 minutes. You will then be moving into the next three exercises, 4-6, again moving from one to another without a break.

4. *Leg Lifts* (in sequence as follows)
Beginning in *Knees to Chest* position (see 3 above), inhale, stretch your arms straight out fully from your sides, and lift both legs together to 60 degrees. Exhale and lower the legs. Continue this for 15 minutes as instructed by the Teacher.

5. Then, continuing on your back, lift the left knee to your chest, holding it with your left arm and hand. Then lift the right leg perpendicular and straight to 90 degrees. Repeat this action with the right leg, up and down, for 1 minute as instructed by the Teacher. Then switch to the opposite leg and repeat the exercise for 1 minute. Repeat this sequence, employing first one leg and then the other, one more time.

6. Quite immediately, stand up, stretching your arms straight above your head and with hand back so that the palms face the ceiling. With the exhale, do a complete *Forward [Front] Bend* laying, or touching, your hands to floor, deep breathing as necessary, and returning to your full standing, arms stretched upward, position. As you do this, apply *Rootlock* [*Mulbandh*] [see Yoga Practice Appendix 2] on the exhales. Repeat this up and down, stretching slow for 2 minutes; then, for 1 more minute, repeat the up and down stretching for 1 minute.

7. *Relax or Meditate* (10-15 mins) / *How to do Savasana* – by Karuna
Come onto your back. Lay your body out on Mother Earth. If you're outdoors, which I highly recommend, lay flat on the

earth, bring your arms by your side, with your palms up. Feel the sun in your solar plexus and inhale from the heart, all the way down from the head to the lowest Chakra. Push your bully full out, and then drop your belly in, up and under, and *pause*. Pause and then *squeeze*—squeeze, squeeze—and then release. Move from the big fat Buddha Belly to a full exhale... Ahhh...! Do this several times until you're melting like Ghee [butter] in the sun. Slowly melt. Dissolve back to zero—"no thing"-ness. Receive the blessing of the sun. Don't use a pillow. That disrupts the energy from your body to your head. Feel the energy running all the way from your Crown Chakra down through your calves, ankles, and toes. Relax your knees, your hips; relax from the tip of *Mata Kundalini* all the way up the spine. Let everything melt into absolute surrender. Relax your jaw, your tongue, your molars. Take three more breaths, inhaling through the back of your Heart and exhaling through the front of your heart. Then take a Yogic Nap for 11 minutes.

Completion Direction from Karuna

Waking from your 11-minute nap, roll onto your side. Pull your knees into your chest and cuddle up into the womb of your own sacred light and breathe—breathe and let go; breathe and let go; breathe and let go. Then bring yourself up again and come seated. You have manifested from a new opportunity and reaped a new abundance. Know that you can experience these gifts *right now*.

12

RECOMMENDATIONS FOR RECIPES AND MUSIC

Yogi Tea: The Essential Drink for Kundalini Yoga Practice

Yogi Tea Recipe. Ingredients: 2 quarts water. 15 cloves (whole). 20 black peppercorns. 3 sticks cinnamon. 20 cardamom pods (split the pods first by gently squashing them with the side of a knife). 8 slices ginger (1/4" thick, no need to peel). 1/2 teaspoon black tea leaves (regular or decaf, or approximately 2 tea bags). Directions: Brew slowly for 3 hours. Share and enjoy!

Favorite Recorded Accompaniments for Kundalini Yoga Practice

Kundalini Morning Aquarian Chants by Jaya Lakshmi & Ananda Das

https://jayalakshmiandanandayogiji.bandcamp.com/album/kundalini-morning-chants

Chant 1. Wah Yantee (Creativity)
Chant 2. Mul Mantra (Inner Truth)
Chant 3. Sat Siri (Beyond Death)
Chant 4. Rakhay Rakanahaar (Protection)
Chant 5. Wahe Guru Wahe Jio (Victory)
Chant 6. Guru Ram Das (Grace & Humility)
Chant 7. Long Time Sun (Completion of Sadhana)
Chant 8. Ra Ma da Sa (Healing)

Chant 9. Ardhas Bhaee (Prayer/Devotion/Miracles)

Chant 10. Ang Sung Wahe Guru / Love like the Sun (Radiance & Oneness)

Albums of Choice

Hari Bhajan Kaur: *Divine Woman (Bhandh Jamee-Ai [Heals the Feminine])*

Snatam Kaur: *Grace (Ray Man Shabad; Long Time Sun)*

Singh Kaur: *Blessings & Crimson 4-6*

Mata Mandir Singh: *Japji: Yoga of Sound Series*

Guru Dass Singh Khalsa: *Flowers in the Rain*

Sirgun Kaur: *The Cosmic Gift, Gobind*

Sat Purkh: *Aisa Naam*

Simran Kaur: *Tantric Har*

Harjinder Singh (aka Sri Nagar Wale): *Best of Bhai Harjinder Singh; Best Shabad Gurbani*

FURTHER PRACTICE

From Karuna:
www.lightonkundalini.com

Introducing

The
LIGHT ON KUNDALINI
YOGA MANUAL

An Inspiration from Karuna
Introduction to the Manual
The Instructional Guides

Foundational Guide [the basic universal Yoga elements used over and over]
Day to Day Guide [all the rest of the Yoga elements ("asanas")]
Sessional Guide ["kriyas" (sequences of asanas)]

Following on her book *Light on Kundalini: Your Lifestyle Guide to Yoga and Awakening*, this is an Instructional Guide for the landscape of Karuna's yoga teachings. In addition to being the standard "go to" guide for working with her Yoga teachings, it parallels the (i) Light on Kundalini website (www.lightonkundalini.com), (ii) Yoga Sessions available on Karuna's LOK App (Apple/Android - https://apps.apple.com/us/app/light-on-kundalini-yoga/id1226594061), (iii) Light on Kundalini YouTube Channel (www.youtube.com/@lightonkundalini), (iv) Karuna's teachings at Sacred U (https://courses.sacredstories.com/pages/meet-karuna) and Humanity's Stream (https://stream.humanitysteam.org/awakening-the-ten-bodies-with-karuna;

https://stream.humanitysteam.org/healing-grief-with-karuna; https://stream.humanitysteam.org/3-minute-meditations-with-karuna; https://stream.humanitysteam.org/81-facets-of-mind-with-karuna), and (v) Yoga Sessions presented hitherto, or in the future, in *Light on Light Magazine* (https://issuu.com/lightonlight), for which Karuna is Host Editor, and all other yoga venues that may be graced by her teachings.

The Guide is illustrated profusely with photographs, featuring Karuna's practice, across all the elements.

From the Introduction

Practicing Yoga is a developmental and evolutionary landscape that works from initial, foundational, understanding to more advanced understanding and practices, all of which build outward and upward—much like limbs and branches of a tree.

In fact, using this metaphor, Patanjali, in the most famous historical work on Yoga—his 2nd Century *Yoga Sutras*—described "The Eight Limbs of Yoga."

Accordingly, this Instructional Guide will work from, first, a "Foundational Guide" which you can think of as the roots and trunk of this tree, and of your own practice. It includes the most basic and fundamental concepts and activities of Yoga practice.

Then follows a detailed "Day to Day Guide" much like the developing branches of your tree, building out through many limbs and branches the entire landscape of yogic practice and understanding.

The third component is an ongoing and developing "Sessional Guide." This is needed because, in building Yogic practice, the various components of Yoga are sequenced in prescribed groupings—called "kriyas"—each of which serves a specific function or has a specific goal. Sequences of these "kriyas" are what make up the "Sessional Guide." You can think of them as all the varieties of foliage and blossom you can create with your growing tree of Yogic practice.

An Inspiration from Karuna

"Whatever that is, I want that!"

That is how I felt after my first Yoga class. I've spent four decades reveling in the intricacies and joy of why that is, and I am not alone.

99% of people told me that I would never be a professional model. Only 1% (Eileen Ford, who helped launch my career) said that I could. I had no mentorship or money. What in me at 19 years old made me listen to the 1% and take that one-way ticket to Paris that resulted in a prolific professional modeling career?

Many people thought I was also crazy for wanting to fly a helicopter. So what was it in me that had me up there alone in a whirling bird taking on winds at will? What countered the fear and the doubt to propel me forward?

At this time, I had an entire family of responsibilities. What gave me the guts to audition while standing on my head for the Bristol Old Vic Theatre School—founded by Laurence Olivier and whose alumni include Olivia Coleman, Daniel Day Lewis, and Anthony Hopkins? What helped me to get accepted and then supported me in getting the lead in *Bartholomew Fair* (1614) by Ben Jonson?

Standing alone in the middle of a decimated home in the Colorado mountains, what gave me the calm, the presence, to handle the destruction, move through the steps of what then needed to be done, and focus on the opportunity of rebuilding, instead of ruminating on what was lost?

It was only the steady reassurance, resounding from my soul, that helped me forward, the "Sat Nam: You and God are one. You are complete. Truth is your essence, your identity. You can do this; you got this; you are what you need right now."

In the words from the scriptures of the Sikh tradition, the wellspring of Kundalini Yoga—from the words of the *Siri Guru Granth Sahib*: "When the God in you, and the human in you are in parallel unisonness, then you are an 11. You have no duality, you have divine vision, and the truth flows from you. You don't have to find anything outside of you. The jewels are all in you—you are rich inside, you have satisfaction and contentment."

A Kundalini Yogi, I connect with my soul and the heart of the universe through the Yogic practices that foster *constant conscious conversation*, or "CCC"—strike more than a pose; take the posture and don't move; let the posture take you. Hold and breathe; choose to listen; hear from your heart, not your ego. What is the posture telling you? Strike up CCC and see!

From the catwalk to the yoga mat, it is going beyond unconscious being or getting wrapped up in "doership", ego, and the mind—through deep self-inquiry, meditation, chanting, asana, and other spiritual practices—that reveals the divine stuff we are made of, awakens us to what our soul has to say, supports us through the intimidation of finding our voice and speaking up, and builds the trust in ourselves that leads us to not only survive but also to thrive in this life.

That's what has brought me to write *Light on Kundalini: Your Lifestyle Guide to Yoga and Awakening* and its companion, *The Light on Kundalini Yoga Manual*, to share the Yogic tools which will foster CCC, awakening and reinforcing your oneness with your soul, your community, and the universe, and giving you the audacity to face the 99% and go with the 1%—to pull through and flourish, like I did.

It is no small statement to make, but Yoga saved my life. It is my deepest wish that it also will help you to live yours. Sat Nam!

KARUNA

ABOUT THE AUTHOR

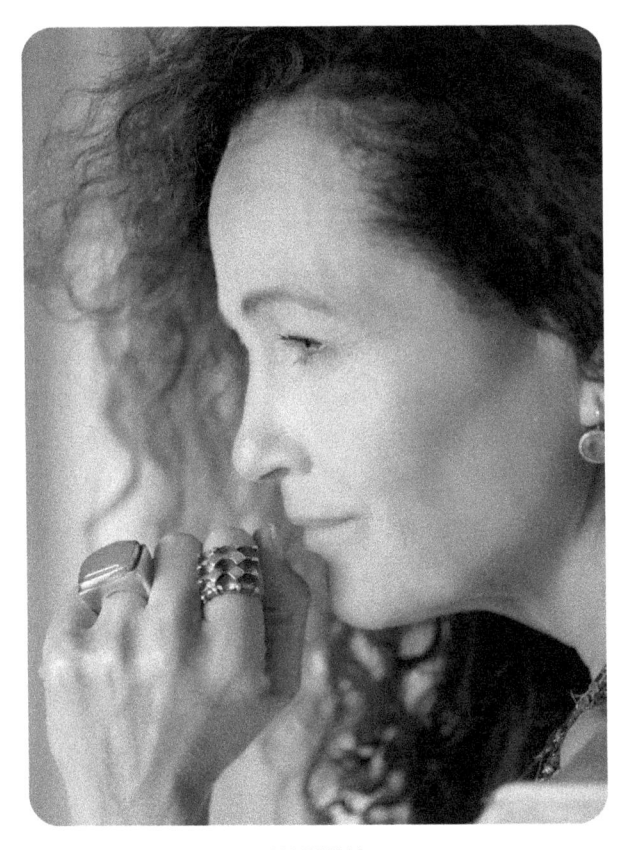

KARUNA

Karuna brings her own unique brand of compassion, enthusiasm, and pure joy to every Kundalini Yoga practice. Based in Boulder, CO, she offers private, one-on-one teachings designed for each individual, holds weekend intensives on varying themes including rebirthings, relationships, women's issues, practicing non-violence, understanding grief, and mastering challenges, and leads special events and retreats all over the world including an annual Reboot Retreat in Costa Rica. Also certified in teaching yoga to children, teenagers, and prenatal moms, Karuna has taught for the Santa Monica/Malibu school system in California, leading classes for second and fourth graders, as well as high school students. She continues to be an Associate Level Trainer in the Aquarian Trainer Academy and facilitates Level One, Level Two, and Level Three teacher training programs and modules in conjunction with Lead Teachers from the Kundalini Research Institute. She also has 15 years of teaching at RallySport Health & Fitness Club, Boulder's oldest health and fitness center, training triathletes and professional swimmers to maintain focus with Mantra and meditation.

Additionally, Karuna practices in the healing arts, which includes a nutritional background in line with Ayurvedic diet and energetic healings in ceremonial and ritual cleansings initiated by the Lakota tradition (in her embodiment as Chanté Eton Wo Wa Gla Ka Win).

Karuna believes "we start from the earth up in any practice, and every practice is reviewed by nature first."

Her personal timeline:

Caroline Diane Boerio (b.-8 years old)
Carrie Pagano (1979-1985)
Caroline Ashley (1985-Present)

A Ford model, Carrie's path to Self discovery began long before she ever took her first Yoga class. Beyond beauty, pouring all her energy and *JOY* into the lens, it was her first discovery of what it meant to offer and hopefully have others feel the pure bliss emanating from her heart.

While studying at the Bristol Old Vic Theatre School in England as Caroline, a classically trained actress (a SAG-AFTRA union member since 1983), she began sharing decades of her own personalized style of Yoga with the young and upcoming students becoming actors, classmates who came to her for her guidance and Yoga practice. She later helped develop The Life Centre's Yoga program in London.

> Chanté Eton Wo Wa Gla Ka Win (1995-Present)
> Karuna (2004-Present)
> Livpreet Kaur (2005-Present)

Karuna continued to find more of herself as she studied Hinduism / Buddhism for seven years in India as well as being apprentice to a Medicine Man of the Lakota Sioux healing tradition. She also received a certificate of ordination as Reverend Caroline Ashley Order of Universal Interfaith-Interspiritual Cleric and Minister and is a member of the Founding Mother's Movement for Planetary Peace and Partnership dedicated to TRUTH, LOVE, and LIGHT.

True to her spiritual name, which means "compassion," Karuna helps her students from all walks of life push beyond self-imposed limits. Her classes are filled with humor, music, and the spirit of transformation.

Karuna's Kundalini Yoga Teachings can be found on her Light on Kundalini website (www.lightonkundalini.com), LOK AP (https://apps.apple.com/us/app/light-on-kundalini-yoga/id1226594061), YouTube Channel (www.youtube.com/@lightonkundalini), Vimeo (https://vimeo.com/ondemand/lightonkundaliniyoga), Instagram (https://www.instagram.com/lightonkundalini/), Facebook (https://www.facebook.com/lightonkundalini/), LinkedIn (https://www.linkedin.com/company/light-on-kundalini/), and X, formerly Twitter (https://twitter.com/LOKundalini/).

Teach.Yoga / Sacred U / Humanity's Stream

Karuna has been featured as a luminary on Teach.Yoga, Sacred U, and Humanity's Stream. You can read more here: https://teach.yoga/karuna/, https://courses.sacredstories.com/pages/meet-karuna, https://stream.humanitysteam.org/healing-grief-with-karuna, https://stream.humanitysteam.org/81-facets-of-mind-with-karuna, https://stream.humanitysteam.org/awakening-the-ten-bodies-with-karuna, and https://stream.humanitysteam.org/3-minute-meditations-with-karuna.

Light on Light Magazine and Media

Karuna was a co-founder of Light on Light Publications and Media (https://www.lightonlight.us/) and its many activities (VoiceAmerica radio, video series, etc.) in 2017. She is Host Editor for its free e-magazines, especially the annual issues published with the International Day of Yoga Committee at the United Nations (https://issuu.com/lightonlight). Karuna is also a host of Light on Light's *Convergence* series on VoiceAmerica (https://www.lightonlight.us/voice-america/) and, given her background in film, represents Light on Light at the ILLUMINATE conscious film festivals, which Light on Light co-sponsors (https://www.illuminatefilmfestival.com/).

What Karuna Wants You to Know

Karuna (*Sanskrit word often translated as "compassion"*) encourages you to find your path and purpose as she has recognized through her own experience how life pokes, provokes, and confronts only to elevate us into our authentic voices and destinies, "waking up, growing up, cleaning up, and showing up" to become a community of enlivened, thriving souls. This book and the accompanying *Light on Kundalini Yoga Manual* are her offerings of support when they find their way into the palms of your hands. At that point, the work is almost 70% done, and these are the practices to guide you to the full and whole 100%. If patience pays, and your politeness and privilege are devotional, you will find yourself heading towards your destiny. Just keep up, and you'll be kept up. Sat Nam!

ABOUT THE CONTRIBUTOR
KURT JOHNSON PHD

Dr. Kurt Johnson, whose Kundalini Yoga training was with Karuna and her Sikh colleagues, is a well-known interfaith and interspiritual leader. Closely associated with interspiritual pioneer Br. Wayne Teasdale for many years, he is the author of *The Coming Interspiritual Age* (2013), a book that followed on Br. Teasdale's *The Mystic Heart: Discovering a Universal Spirituality in the World's Religions*. Br. Teasdale, Kurt, and others co-founded Interspiritual Dialogue (ISD) (http://www.isdna.org/) in 2002, two years before Br. Teasdale's transition. ISD then became the parent of Light on Light Publications and Media (https://www.lightonlight.us/) and its many activities (VoiceAmerica radio, video series etc.) co-founded in 2017 and now including Kurt, Karuna, Dr. Robert Atkinson, Shannon and David Winters, Nomi Naeem and Chamatkara (Sandra Simon). Kurt and colleagues founded https://www.interspirituality.com/ in 2015. Kurt, along with Karuna, host Light on Light's *Convergence* series on VoiceAmerica. Light on Light's books are an imprint of Sacred Stories (https://sacredstories.com/).

Also a scientist with a PhD in Evolution and Ecology (and author of over 200 scientific articles and seven technical books), Kurt is author or co-author of influential and award-winning popular-books: *Our Moment of Choice* (2020) (Gold Nautilus, COVR and Living Now Awards), *Nabokov's Blues* (2000) and *Fine Lines* (2015) (Brian Boyd Prize, 2019). Kurt served on the faculty of New York's One Spirit Interfaith Seminary for 15 years and, for 25 years, was also associated there with the American Museum of Natural History. Active today in numerous global change Impact Networks, Kurt is Coordinator of the Synergy Circles of the Evolutionary Leaders (https://www.evolutionaryleaders.net/synergycircles), part of the

Core Team for the Holomovement (https://www.holomovement.net/), a co-visioner of https://unity.earth/ & https://oneworld.earth/, and member of the https://www.prosocial.world/ Stewardship Council.

A former monastic, Kurt is ordained, or certified, in five religious traditions, is a member or founder of the Evolutionary Leaders, Association of Transformational Leaders, international Contemplative Alliance, Gaiafield and Subtle Activism Networks, Self Care to Earth Care network, UN NGO Committee on Spirituality, Values and Global Concerns, NGO Forum 21 Institute, the UN Committee for International Yoga Day, and is President of the Friends of the Institute of Noetic Sciences. He has received the Synergy Super Star award from the Evolutionary Leaders, the Lifetime Achievement Award from the Visioneers, and God's Partner award from One Spirit Interfaith Seminary in New York City.

ACKNOWLEDGMENTS

Because this book culminates my life's work to date, there are so many people to acknowledge and thank. Accordingly, the order here cannot be taken as reflecting any kind of rank. I am indebted to them all.

Let's start with my family (or families!) who have played such important roles from the very beginning. My mother, Diana Pagano–always a mirror to me–a celebrated opera singer, the great beauty of her voice and her being, the inspiration for me always to be myself. My biological dad, Chuck Boerio, a true "mountain man," always a force in my life, who gave the gifts of humor, rugged physicality, and (as collector of historical memorabilia) an appreciation for the delicacy of "little things." My second dad, Sam Pagano, anchor of the professional sports lineage of my family who, with my brothers, brought the messages of hardwork, fitness, and excellence.

My well-known brothers, both NFL coaches–Chuck and John Pagano–who have always entwined their lives with mine, not only with the values of excellence that come with sport but also their care for multiple humanitarian and charitable activities.

Loving memories as well of my Grandmother, Suzanna Fusek, a Slovakian refugee smuggled into this country for her own safety during the World Wars' desparate times; and my dearest Uncle Joe, Joseph Domko, III. Their love and care for me I have never forgotten.

My beloved departed sister, Catherine Pagano, who features so prominently in this book. Along with all I impart about her within these pages, she is truly always with me. And, my sisters, Constance Dennerline and Jennifer Pagano, with whom, blessed with our long years of shared sisterhood, have added so much to my life.

Of course, my children, Emily Laura Ashley and Tomas Oliver Ashley, whose stories stand side by side with mine within this book—no words could sum that up. They have been a joy and fulfillment to my life, at every stage of their own growing and maturing into the wonderful adults they are today. And to their beloved spouses, Michelle Yildiz-Ashley and Thomas Caprarella, who have so well continued our legacy of Family.

My extended and historical family—the Ashleys of the legendary fashion world: Sir Bernard Ashley (an incredibly rich relationship that I will always hold deep in my heart, forever grateful!) and Laura Ashley (my mentor to this day to bring forth the importance of the Divine Feminine and for women to be respected and recognized). I will always be grateful for my irreplaceable experiences within that iconic fashion culture. I married their son, David Ashley, and we birthed two beautiful children that have been a source of devotion and resilience for me all my life.

My pantheon of friends—I don't know where to begin. Pamela Hanson, author of the heartfelt upfront Personal Note to me herein, has been a beloved companion since "discovering" me for my modeling career when I was nineteen years old (her then companion, Bernard Grant, took my first photos and was so kind with this amateur). So many of my early stories herein are from that life-shaping growth period of my story, and beloved Pamela has always been there, sharing courage, inner faith, trust, and friendship for which I am forever grateful.

In the spiritual community, again, so many prized and dear friends as I have grown and prospered: Hari Kaur Khalsa, a soul sister on my Kundalini Yoga path, her counsel on trusting the Guru and her unwavering friendship and reliability as an amazing sister on the path. Swami Prakashananda, a teacher of the divine in the softest way of how we learn from ourselves as we stay on the path. And, my dear friend Diane Marie Williams who has supported me throughout and nurtured the integrating of my skill sets, the late Philip Hellmich, the beloved peace ambassador for The Shift Network, and Jeff Vander Clute who helped us coin the phrase "Light on Light."

Of course, *so* central to my life—Sadhvi Bhagawati Saraswati and the revered master, H.H. Swami Chidanand Saraswatiji of Parmarth Niketan Ashram, Rishikesh, India. Sadhviji who has so kindly written the Afterword to this book, and Swamiji who, for whatever reason, has taken such a personal interest in my life and so movingly hosting the Puja for my father and the scattering of his ashes in the sacred Ganga.

For deep friendship and years of collegial work in the global Yoga community, Denise Scotto, Chair of the International Day of Yoga Committee at the United Nations, another devotee of the Parmarth Niketan community, who has written the Foreword to this book—we have many more shared journeys ahead!

Deep thanks to Isak Hanold, my nearly life-long collaborator for photography, video, and film—not only a great filmmaker and director but an unwavering and always reliable friend. And, to Teg Ranjeet, a student who has stepped up so creatively for creation of my newsletter and my LOK App. Thanks as well to John McClosky, who across this entire journey has been my legal counsel and Trustee, always diligent to serve my best interests and all of those around me.

As this book has progressed, dear friend Melanie Paykos who came forward to simultaneously design this book and its companion Yoga Manual, bringing to this production the gifted designer Henriqué Teixiera, further adding to the amazing grace of this creative process.

My editor, and friend and collaborator, Chamatkara (Sandra Simon) of Light on Light Press—another lineage holder with Sw. Prakashananda in the Sacred Feet Yoga lineage of Sw.

Shraddhananda (aka Dr. Sonya Jones). What a super-sweet angelic editor I landed, who has understood so deeply all of the intended nuances of this book. I am forever grateful.

Finally, Dr. Robert Atkinson and Dr. Kurt Johnson, also Managing Editors of Light on Light Press. Bob not only has participated with this book but also enjoys Kundalini Yoga with his radiant presence. Kurt, with whom I have now worked in the spiritual community for over a dozen years (and P.S., *no one* introduced us), has been part of both this book's creation, and its companion Yoga Manual, from the beginning. As the book recounts, it began with several weeks of discussions on my back veranda under the majestic peaks on the backside of the Continental Divide. I spoke and dictated the contents of this book, and he recorded. How we got from over 300 pages of notes from those discussions to this book is truly a miracle, likely reflecting the mind- and soul-melds that seem to be happening in so many places in the amazing and also incredibly challenging historical times of which we are all a part.

MESSAGE FROM THE PUBLISHER

Light on Light Press produces enhanced content books spotlighting the sacred ground upon which all religious and wisdom traditions intersect; it aims to stimulate and perpetuate engaged interspiritual and perennial wisdom dialogue for the purpose of assisting the dawning of a unitive consciousness that will inspire compassionate action toward a just and peaceful world.

We are delighted to publish *Light on Kundalini: Your Lifestyle Guide to Yoga and Awakening* because it is a one-of-a-kind guidebook to yogic lifestyle and practices, offering a unique perspective on a most important Awakening journey. This book brings bright light to the world, helping one find the Way to the True Self—*and* the blessing of deep and authentic relationships with companions on the Path.

Light on Kundalini demystifies, and makes accessible, all the aspects of Yoga—Kundalini, meditation, grace, Sadhana, Ayurveda, and the Kriyas—lovingly guiding one along that Perennial Path that is at once unknown, but yet well-traveled. Karuna's personal story, style, and expertise enlighten the Way—fashioning a deeply engaging and detailed roadmap, a daily companion for well-being and happiness in finding one's unique path to Ultimate Destiny.

We consider this to be a groundbreaking book in the breadth and depth of its clarity on the Kundalini Yoga landscape—from the Chakras to a Unitive Cosmology, the gift of community, seeing in others what they can't see in themselves, and experiencing the Divine in "every-day" life. It uniquely offers a welcoming and supportive "Wisdom Village," not just to visit but also as a Home to return to daily—to take a break in, relax and reflect, and be nurtured by communion with our Deepest Nature.

We welcome *Light on Kundalini* in taking its place among our other books that tell our timeless, universal story in which "union" (Yoga) is the very center—and the embracing periphery—of all things.

Managing Editors
Kurt Johnson PhD
Robert Atkinson PhD
Nomi Naeem MA
Chamatkara (Sandra Simon)

Printed in the USA
CPSIA information can be obtained
at www.ICGtesting.com
CBHW051442261124
18035CB00012B/627